Yoga—
A Path for Happy Life

Yoga—
A Path for Happy Life

Manan Aggarwal

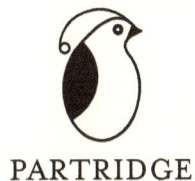

PARTRIDGE

To order additional copies of this book, contact
Partridge India
000 800 10062 62
orders.india@partridgepublishing.com

www.partridgepublishing.com/india

Contents

An important message to my readers:

The Asanas and Pranayams in this book should not be attempted without the supervision of an experienced teacher or prior experience. The ideas expressed in this book should not be used to diagnose, prescribe, treat, cure or prevent any disease, illness, or individual health problems. Consult your health practitioners for individual health care. The information provided within this book is believed to be accurate based on the personal experience of the author but the reader is responsible for consulting with their own health professional before changing the diet or starting an exercise program. This book is an humble initiative to share benefit of Yoga with society without any motive of profit making. We shall not be liable for any direct, indirect, incidental, special, consequential, or punitive injuries resulting from the use of this book.

About the Author

Born in Delhi in 1999, Manan Aggarwal, a high school student, shares his journey into the world of Yoga which had changed his life immensely. In his book "Yoga – A Path for Happy Life", he tries to covers the different aspects of Yoga covering a wide range of Asanas, Pranayams. An active Yoga participant for the past few years, he has come to appreciate the metamorphic changes which Yoga had brought into his life. Slowly but steadily, he wishes to spread this appreciation further and with this book, he has taken his first step.

Dedicated to all my revered Gurus'

Preface

It is thanks to the persistent encouragement of my Gurus' and family that this book is now achieved – for alone I would have repeatedly faltered by losing heart without their support and assurance.

Yoga is a practical science which deals with the physical as well as phychological aspect of human being. Yoga is a precious legacy of Ancient Indian culture science. Yoga is the foundation stone of happy and healthy life. It ensures not only physical well being but infuses a sense of tranquillity, balances physiological and psychological functioning with nature. This infusion does not come in a day or two but penetrates slowly and gradually from our consciousness to our unconscious one. Yoga embraces us as whole.

This book describes *simply* but in great detail the 46 Asanas (Postures) and 5 Pranayama's (Breathing disciplines), providing a comprehensive introduction to yoga. It describes the techniques for 46 Asanas with the aid of photographs and it also covers 5 Pranayama's with the aid of the photographs.

All the ancient commentaries have stressed upon the importance of working under the direction of a Guru (Master), and although my experience proves the wisdom of this rule, I have endeavoured with all humility in this book to guide the reader to a correct and safe method of mastering these Asanas and Pranayams.

I am sincerely grateful to my all Gurus. I am highly indebted to my father for introducing me to this world of Yoga. He has been a pillar of strength and support throughout my journey, so thanks Dad!

I express my sincere gratitude to Mr Dev and Mr Raj for their personal supervision and interest in taking innumerable photographs for me and for placing the resources of the studio at my disposal.

Manan Aggarwal

Introduction

Yoga essentially means, union of the individual soul with the Universal Spirit. Yoga is an Indian ancient legacy of knowledge and wisdom. Though to many, yoga is only one form of physical exercise involving twist, turn, stretch, and breathe in different ways, but these are actually only fraction of profound science of unfolding of various aspects of the human body, mind and soul that deciphers code of happiness.

The science of Yoga is culmination of various aspect of Life – Gyan (philosophy), Bhakti (devotion), Karma (action) and Raja Yoga (mind control). Raja Yoga balances and unifies all aspects of life in the form Yoga Asana. There is greater emphasis on the inner experience of meditation, for the well-being of mind and other hidden elements of human existence. When one is in harmony with oneself, life becomes calmer, happier and more fulfilled.

The greatest thing about yoga is that it embraces all body structures irrespective of their age without any side effects, thereby connecting you to the nature. You begin working on the external physical alignment and mechanics of the yoga postures till it reaches to your inner being in the asana. Yoga is not alien to us but we can see that its many asana are simply mimicking of natural posture, animal forms like cat stretch, monkey stretch, crocodile stretch, dog stretch, spider stretch, fish stretch, cobra stretch and likewise many others that strengthens various parts of our body in more than our limited ways. Yoga, in many ways, is "A Path for Happy Life."

This has also increased the respect that that I have for myself respect for others. I feel this stems a lot from the self-confidence I found through yoga. Before yoga, I was an impatient person, snapping at even the slightest pause. If I have an idea or goal, I want it done then and right then. Yoga has changed that. Just like I couldn't master all the best poses in yoga at first, I couldn't complete all my goals at once either. I was patient enough to learn to listen to my body and let it guide me on its own terms. I had to wait. The things and goal that I had before, the person I aspire to be are still the same today too but I am dealing them with patience, time and practice.

Remembering that every little detail forms us into the person that we are right now. My yoga journey is far from over and that's what is most exciting, finding out what is next in store and also the same can be said for my life journey. I don't feel anxious about the future, I can go on and embrace it more with collective ease. That means a lot to me going forward.

Yoga And Its Objective

Some one said "What we KNOW, is SCIENCE, and what we do not, is GOD"

Yoga is part of the such science, that evolved many years ago when there were no Universities, laboratories or any award to appreciate their contributions to human civilization. Yoga evolved by combined efforts of many famous as well as unnamed ancient sages and rishis (dedicated students).

Yoga is that part of science which integrates harmonical functioning of various other parts of science(Physics, Chemical science, medical science, psychological science, cosmical science etc. It's goal is to achieve peace, bliss and happiness, which starts from person itself.

Maharishi (great rishi) PATANJALI was the one, who gave knowledge of YOGA to human mankind. He was a great Philosopher and Physician as well..

According to Patanjali, Yoga is culmination all faculties of the mind with physical body. According to Yoga body, functions as per codified instructions of minds. No physical body problem can be solved in isolation but is to be treated from root for a wholesome cure. Yoga has this ability to offer a wholesome solutions with no side effects on body or environment. Yoga deals with body, mind and whole universe on micro as well as macro level.

Yoga means "to join" in Sanskrit (one of the Indian language used in ancient India). Yoga, being evolved on Indian soil, emphasizes on spirituality. It guide us to connect individual soul (Atma) with Supreme Soul (Parmatma – GOD). Yoga follows doctrine of peace for all. It harmonizes biotic and abiotic (sun, moon, air and nature) environment leading to wholesome integrated healthy and happy mankind full of Infinite Bliss, Supreme Peace, Infinite Knowledge and unbroken Joy.

Yoga trains mind to liberate from senseless mundane control. It helps us to communicate with nature. It inhibits all sorts of pain(physical as well as emotional), which are root cause of unhappiness, anxiety, poor health and restlessness. Indian Philosphy believes in Birth-Rebirth cycle. According to Indian Philosphy our ultimate Bliss is achieved when one gets liberated from this cycle. Yoga bestows this liberation from the rebirth cycle.

Among many factors of Yoga, self-training and study and practice of different actions are crucial in achievement of ultimate goal of Yoga - happiness and bliss.

Yoga is omnipresent in our all actions and thoughts. Yoga is wholesome inclusive of all micro as well as macro influence. It is all round development of human body well knit with mind and soul.

According to Yoga science we, human beings are embodied with five factors, which are responsible for our physical and mental problems. Yoga helps to treat these factors.. The five afflictions are:

IGNORANCE

EGO

ATTACHMENT

JEOLOUSY

ANGER

Ignorance is root of rest of four factors. Ignorance leads to ego. And wherever is ego one can find rest of three factors strongly attached.

The Yoga believer and follower should first try to control these five factors. One should have strong belief in the efficacy of his Yoga practices. Strong belief stimulates the cosmic energy to flow through Yoga practices in the body. Once cosmic energy starts flowing in the body, there will be abundance of energy, focus and concentration etc.

Therefore, to achieve energy, focus, concentration and the practice of Yoga, one must have abundance of patience, strong will, dedication, commitment and perseverance. Take a dive in concentration. Merge the soul in the universal spirit – God. Allow soul and mind to be absorbed in universal spirit. Allow the whole body upto cellular level be submerged in the idea of God. This is the only key to happiness and blessed health. Great sages and saints in ancient time had practiced Yoga in this way only. What they have achieved, can be achieved by others also. This is the timeless Law of nature.

A. SURYA NAMASKAR

Surya Namaskar is an Yogic expression to pay tribute to the Sun. Sun is one of the Hindu Gods since ancient times. Hindu philosophy treats all components of nature with great regard as they believe that each component contributes in the welfare of human being.

Surya Namaskar facilitates our body for Asanas. Though it can be done at any time of day as people have very hectic schedule but if choice is there, then early morning, when sun rises, is best time.

There is a rule of yoga that its practices should be done with empty stomach.

Surya Namaskar tones and heals the body and freshes the mind.

Surya Namaskar when coupled with speed, proves an intensive workout and enables to shed extra harmful fats.

Surya Namaskar is a sequence of twelve Asanas. It co-ordinates body, breath and mind together –leading to meditation mode. Twelve Asanas of Surya Namaskar relate to the 12 zodiac signs also.

- ### Namaskar Asana

1. On sunrise, choose a clean outdoor place
2. Now stand straight facing sun in happy and relaxed mood.
3. While standing take care that feet should be in attentive position with least distance between two foots and no bending of knees.
4. Feet should be positioned side to side
5. Now join your hands in saluted pose.
6. Now bring saluted hands close to centre of chest with fingers pointing towards your face as shown in picture.

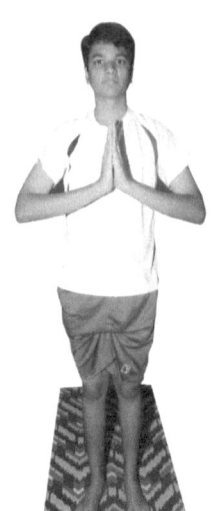

- ### Urdhavhastana Asana

1. When one completes namaskar asana then breath in air slowly and bend towards your back.
2. Now open your hands and take them first towards sky and then towards your back as shown in picture.
3. While doing so, eyes will face sky. Enjoy!

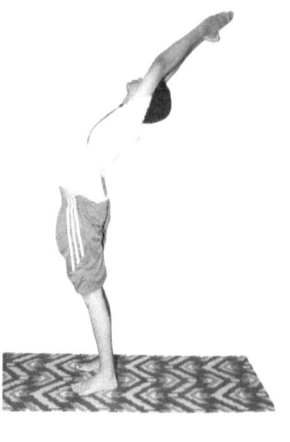

- ### Paadhasta Asana

1. Now breathe out slowly and make reverse movement of your hand and body till body is standing straight with hands up.
2. We will continue movement of our arms and body in forward direction till hands touch sole of your feet left and right respectively.
3. In this process make your head to touch your knee without bending them as shown in picture.

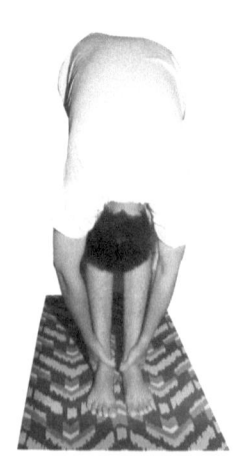

- ### Ashvasanchalan Asana

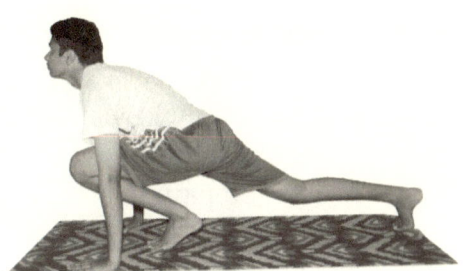

1. Now bend down and move slowly your hands on both sides of body while maintaining body balance with your both palms on the ground.
2. Now move your left foot backward so that it stretches to its maximum straight line touching down ground only with inverted toes while right knee will bend in such a way that it will be facing to your face without any change in position of right foot.
3. Eyes should be watching upwards towards sky while retaining inhaled air as shown in picture

- ### Parvata Asana

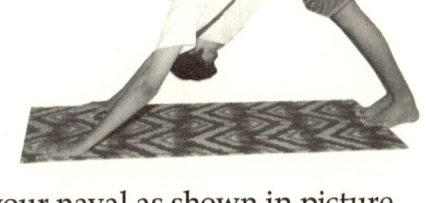

1. Now while breathing move right foot also backward.
2. Keep neck and hand should be in between your both hands.
3. Now lift your hips and back upwards.
4. Now bend your head inwards such a way that your eyes should be focussed towards your naval as shown in picture.

- ### Ashtangnamana Asana – Sashtangasana

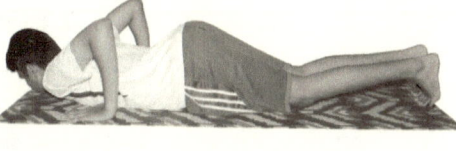

1. Now breathe out and let it normalize.
2. While stabilizing hand knee and feet on ground touch your chest and chin also to ground.
3. The hips and abdomen remain raised as shown in picture.

- **Bhujang Asana**

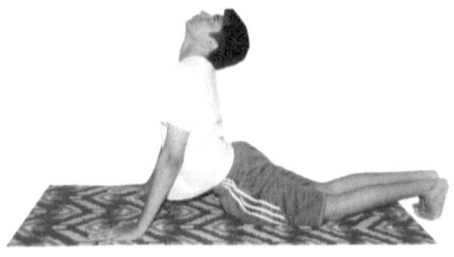

1. While inhaling lift your chest upwards and slowly make hand straight standing on ground on palms.
2. Make sure both Feet should be fully stretched straight and close together.
3. Now lower part of body till naval should touch the ground.
4. While doing so eyes should be focussed towards sky as shown in picture.

- **Parvata Asana (Reverse)**

1. Now breathe out and lift your hips upward while keeping neck and head in between hands.
2. Now lift thighs and back collectively upwards.
3. Bend your head down in such a way that eyesight should be towards your naval as shown in picture.

- **Ashvasanchalan Asana - Reverse**

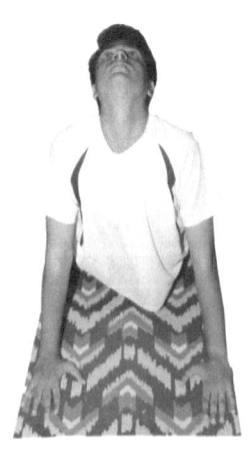

1. Now bend down and take slowly your hands on both sides of chest while maintaining body balance with your both palms on the ground.
2. Now move slowly left foot and take it backward so that it stretches to its maximum straight touching ground only with inverted toes while right knee will bend in such a way that it will be facing to your face without any

change in position of right foot. The heel of right foot should touch ground.

3. Eyes should be watching upwards towards sky while retaining inhaled air as shown in picture.

- ## Paadhasta Asana - Reverse

1. Now breathe out air slowly
2. And bring your hands from back to forward bending till hands touches sole of your feet left and right respectively.
3. Now try to touch knee with your head.
4. Take care not to bend knees as shown in picture.

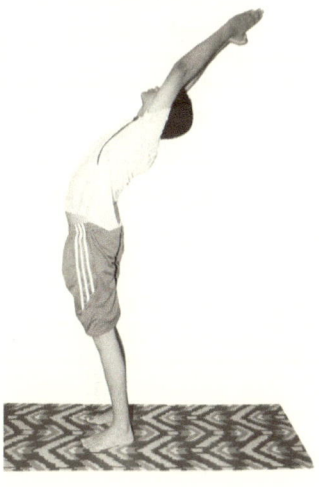

- ## Urdhavhastasana - Reverse

1. Now bend towards backward slowly
2. Breathe in air slowly
3. Now open joined saluted posed hands and take them away upward towards your back without bending elbows keeping your head in the centre of arms...
4. Now stop breathing for a while and watch sky in front of your eyes peacefully.
5. Now bend back also backward as much as possible as shown in picture.

- **Namaskar Asana - Reverse**

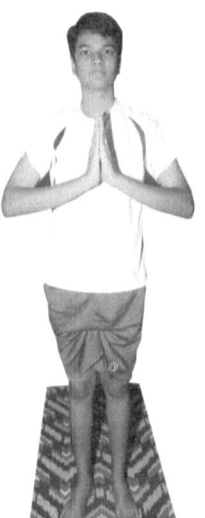

1. Now move back to sun facing position while normal breathing.
2. Make heels, toes and knee should be close together from side to side.
3. Make join your hands side by side with fingers facing chin.
4. Now bring joined hand saluted pose close to centre of chest as shown in picture.

BENEFITS:

➤ Surya Namaskar postures are energising, meditative and relaxing. The whole body feels energised.
➤ It revitalize stomach, small intestine, heart and lungs.
➤ It Provides flexibility to back and spine, smoothens blood circulation, prevents hair greying, hair fall, dandruff and enhances overall hair growth
➤ It keeps skin ailments, stress, anxiety, lethargy and depression at bay.
➤ It stabilises the hormonal secretion and infuses mental and physical freshness leading to happiness.

PRECAUTION:

➤ If one is ill or sick, it should not be done.
➤ It should be done under supervision of experience yoga teacher.
➤ It should be done in relaxed environment.
➤ It should be done in earliest part of the day preferably at the dawn of the day(sunrise).
➤ Empty stomach is recommended.
➤ Avoid any jerk or force during or in assuming any pose.

B. CHANDRA NAMASKAR

Like Surya Namaskar, Chandra Namaskar is also Yogic expression of tribute to Chand (Moon). Moon is one of the Hindu Gods since ancient times. Hindu philosophy treats all components of nature with great regard as they believe that each component contributes in the welfare of human being. According to ancient Indian text moon is the source of immortality. Moon is never been same in fixed phase. It changes daily. It's different phases have varying impacts on the earth.

Although, the Chandra Namaskar can be done at any time, but as the name suggests it is most effective when done in moon-night.

There is a rule of yoga that its practices should be done with empty stomach.

The Chandra namaskar is sequence of fourteen Asanas. The fourteen Asanas of Chandra Namaskar are related to it's fourteen lunar phases.

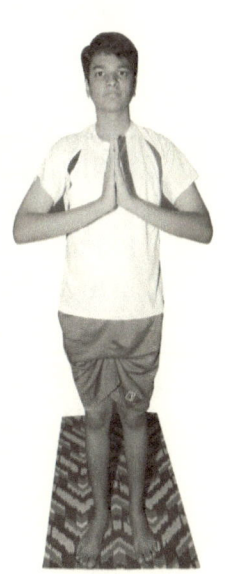

- **Namaskar Asana**

  1. On moonrise, choose a clean outdoor place
  2. Now stand straight facing moon in happy and relaxed mood.

3. While standing take care that feet should be in attentive position with least distance between two foots and no bending of knees.
4. Feet should be positioned side to side
5. Now join your hands in saluted pose.
6. Now bring saluted hands close to centre of chest with fingers pointing towards your face as shown in picture.

- ## Hasta Uttanasana - (2 nd Cyclic Movement)

1. Bring the arms to shoulder width apart.
2. Bring them over head and raise the torso with spine straight.
3. Bend backward slowly
4. Inhale air slowly.
5. Open the saluted hands and take them away upward towards your back without bending elbows keeping your head in the centre of your arms
6. Hold breathing for a while and watch sky in front of your eyes peacefully.
7. Bend back backward as much as possible as shown in picture.

- ## Paadhasta/ Utanasana Asana - (3rd Cyclic Movement)

1. Exhale air slowly
2. Bring your hands from back to forward bending till hands touches sole of your feet left and right respectively.
3. Try to touch your knee with your head.

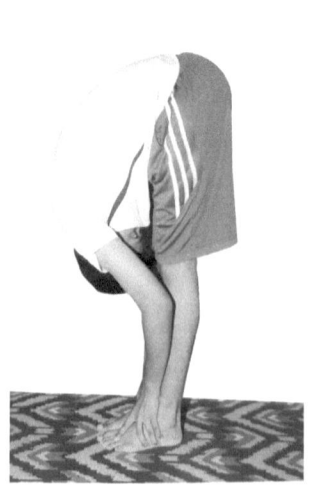

4. Take care not to bend knees as shown in picture.
5. Keep body relaxed. Do not strain any body parts.

- **Ardh-Chandra Asana (4th Cyclic Movement)**

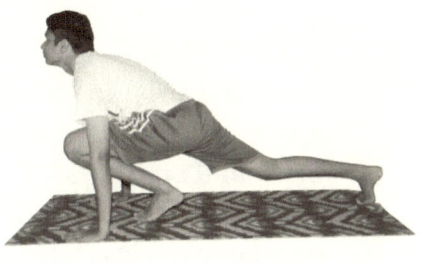

1. Raise the hands, and stretch both arms over the head keeping them shoulder width apart.
2. Arch the back look up, raising the chin as shown in picture.

- **Adhomukha Svanasana/ Parvata Asana (5th Cyclic Movement)**

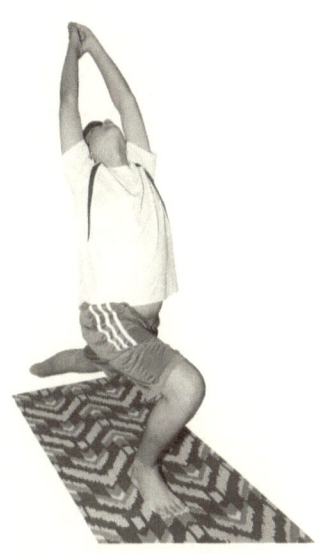

1. While exhaling take right foot also back.
2. Bring the palms on the floor.
3. Neck and hand should be in between your both hands.
4. Lift your hips and back upwards.
5. Lengthening through the spine, bringing the shoulders toward the ankles.
6. Bend your head in such a way that your eyes should be focussed towards your naval as shown in picture.

- **Ashtangnamana Asana (Sashtangasana) (6th Cyclic Movement)**

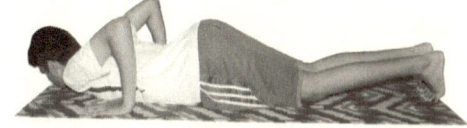

1. Exhale and normalize breathe.

2. Coming onto your toes, simultaneously lower the knees, chin, and chest to the floor. The hips and abdomen remain raised as shown in picture.

- **Bhujang Asana(7ᵗʰ Cyclic Movement)**

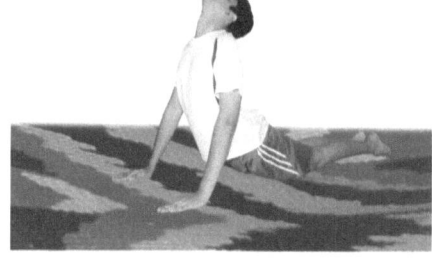

1. While inhaling lift your chest upwards and slowly make hand straight standing on ground on palms.
2. Both feet should be fully stretched and close together.
3. Lower part of body till naval should touch the ground.
4. But eyes should be focussed upwards towards sky as shown in picture.

- **Adhomukha Svanasana/ Parvata Asana (Reverse) - (8ᵗʰ Cyclic Movement)**

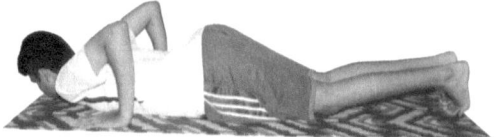

1. Perform the 6ᵗʰ Cyclic movement again.

- **9ᵗʰ Cyclic Movement**

1. While exhaling take right foot also back.
2.   Bring the palms on the floor.
3. Neck and hand should be in between your both hands.
4. Lift your hips and back upwards.
5. Lengthening through the spine, bringing the shoulders toward the ankles.
6. Bend your head in such a way that your eyes should be focus as shown in picture.

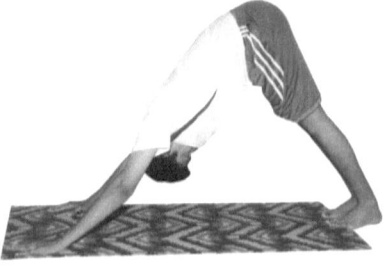

- **Ashvasanchalan asana (Reverse)- 10th Cyclic Movement**

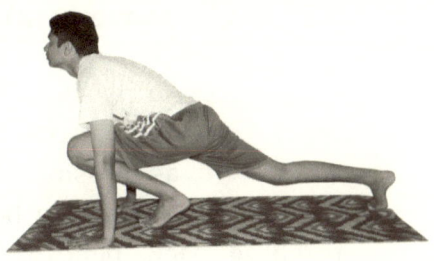

1. Inhale and bend down and take slowly your hands on both sides of chest while maintaining body balance with your both palms on the ground.
2. Lift slowly left foot and take it backward so that it stretches to its maximum straight touching back ground only with inverted toes while right knee will bend in such a way that it will be facing to your face without any change in position of right foot making back little arch shape.
3. Eyes should be watching upwards towards sky while retaining inhaled air as shown in picture.

- **Ardh-Chandra Asana - (11th Cyclic Movement)**

1. Raise your hands and stretch both arms over the head keeping them shoulder width apart.
2. Arch the back look up, raising the chin (Same as 4th Cyclic movement).

- **Utanasana / Paadhasta Asana (12th Cyclic Movement)**

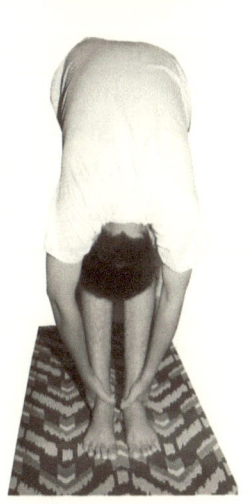

1. Bring the right foot next to the left, and straighten the knees.
2. Bring the crown of the head towards the floor. (Same as cycle 3)

- **Hasta Uttanasana/Urdhavhastasana (13ᵗʰ Cyclic Movement)**

  1. Keeping the arms shoulder width apart, raise the torso with spine as straight as possible. 2. Bring the hands up over the head, and reaching back, bending slightly. (Same as step 2)

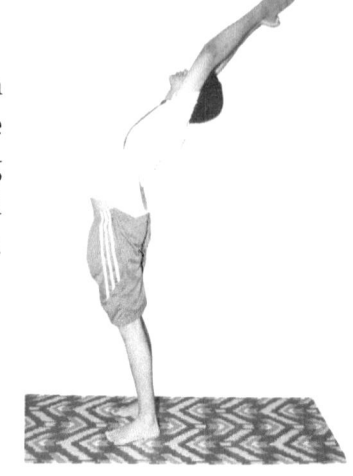

- **Pranam Asana (Salutation Pose) (14ᵗʰ Cyclic Movement)**

  1. Bring the palms together in front of the chest centre. (Same as step 1)

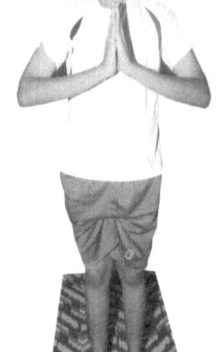

BENEFITS:

  - It helps in channelizing the lunar energy; which has cool, relaxing, and creative.
  - It stretches the spine, hamstrings, and backs of legs; strengthens leg, arm, back, and stomach muscles.
  - Like all other yoga practices, it is important that you learn Chandra Namaskar under proper supervision and guidance.

PRECAUTION:

- ➢ It should be done under supervision of experience yoga teacher.
- ➢ If one is ill or sick, it should not be done.
- ➢ It should be done in relaxed environment.
- ➢ It should be done in the evening at the moonrise.
- ➢ Empty stomach is recommended.
- ➢ Avoid any jerk or force during or in assuming any pose.
- ➢ Breathing Should Be Natural.
- ➢ Any one suffering from chronic disease should also avoid it.

C. YOGA ASANAS (RAJ YOG)

One of the many benefits of practising yoga Asanas is the fact that it allows us to slip into meditation effortlessly. Meditation being one of the important aspects of Yoga, it's preferable that we should sit for meditation after practising Yoga asanas and pranayama.

1. KONA SANA 1 (One arm Angle pose)

KONA =ANGLE; ASANA = POSE/POSTURE

Steps:

* ❖ Relax and stand straight with feet wide apart of hip width distance with arms alongside the body.
* ❖ Inhale and slowly lift the left arm up keeping fingers pointed upwards facing the sky.
* ❖ Exhale and now bend towards the right slowly first from the spine. Do the same with your left side.
* ❖ Now relax a while and repeat all steps with the right arm.

BENEFITS:

* ➢ It helps in toning the sides of the body and spine.
* ➢ It helps in toning of arms, legs and vital organs.
* ➢ Helpful in relieving back pain.
* ➢ It enhances the flexibility of the spine.
* ➢ It relieves from constipation.
* ➢ Helpful for people suffering from sciatica.

PRECAUTIONS:

➢ Spondylitis patient should avoid this pose.
➢ No jerk or force should be applied while doing asana.
➢ It should be done under supervision and guidance of trained Yoga teacher.

2. KONA SANA 2 (Two arm Angle pose)

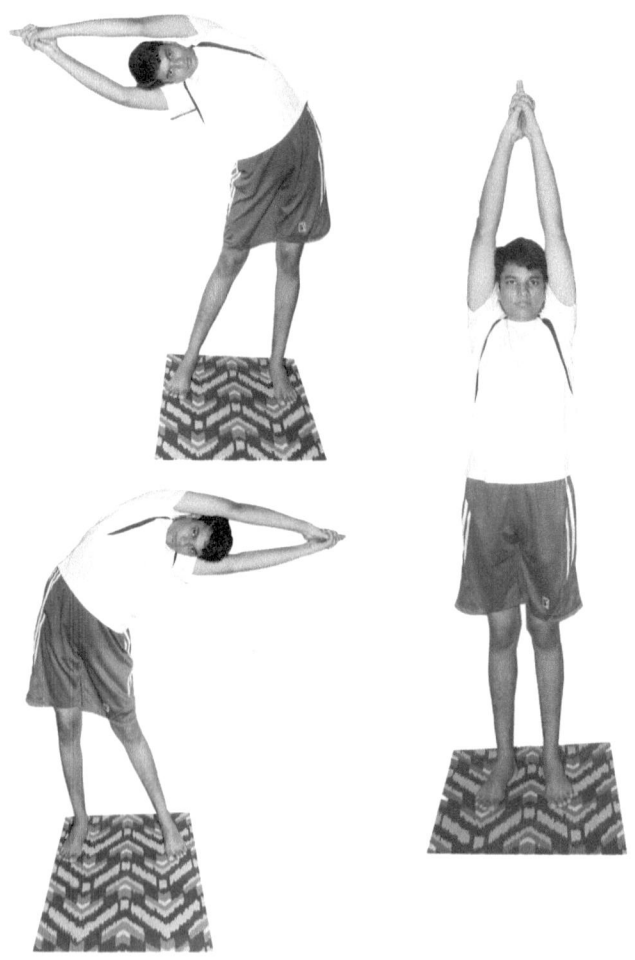

Kona =Angle; Asana = Pose/Posture

Steps:

- ❖ Relax and stand with feet wide apart maximum as per body convenience. Maintain the balance on feet.
- ❖ Inhale and slowly lift arms over the head and join the palms together, interlacing the fingers to form a steeple position. The arms should touch your ears as shown in picture.
- ❖ Exhale out, bend towards the right keeping elbow straight. Maintain your balance on feet and move your pelvis towards the left.
- ❖ Hold this posture as long as you can with body's comfort. Relax a while. Inhale, exhale deep with gentle breaths
- ❖ Now move your upper body including hand in reverse direction till you restore straight standing position while inhaling as shown in picture.
- ❖ Slowly bring the arms down while exhaling.
- ❖ Similarly repeat all steps using the other side.

BENEFITS:

- ❖ It stretches and tones the sides of the body and the spine.
- ❖ It tones the arms, legs, and other vital organs.

3. SHAVA ASANA

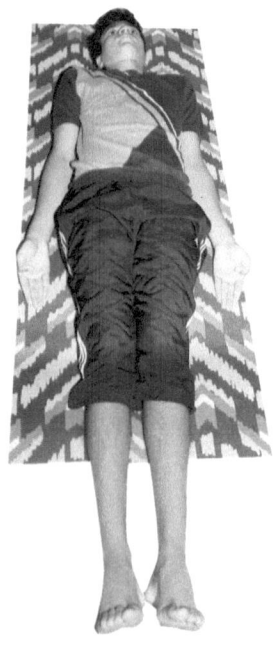

SHAVA – LIFELESS BODY; ASANA - POSE

Steps:

- ❖ This is most easy and relaxed Asana.
- ❖ You lay down in sleeping pose in such a way that your face, abdomen and straight leg facing upwards towards sky.
- ❖ Make your both arms comfortable on both sides of your body.

❖ Your arms should be laid straight with open palms facing sky as shown in picture.
❖ Now declutter your mind from any thought and allow your body relax leisurely.
❖ Now this is holidaying phase for your all body parts.
❖ Maintain your normal breathing. In this process take care not to sleep.
❖ Stay in the pose for a while. When you feel complete relaxation, slowly and gently get up.

BENEFITS:

➢ It heals upto cellular level, bursting stress and restlessness.
➢ It refreshes the whole body.
➢ It normalizes blood pressure and checks insomnia.

4. NATRAJA ASANA

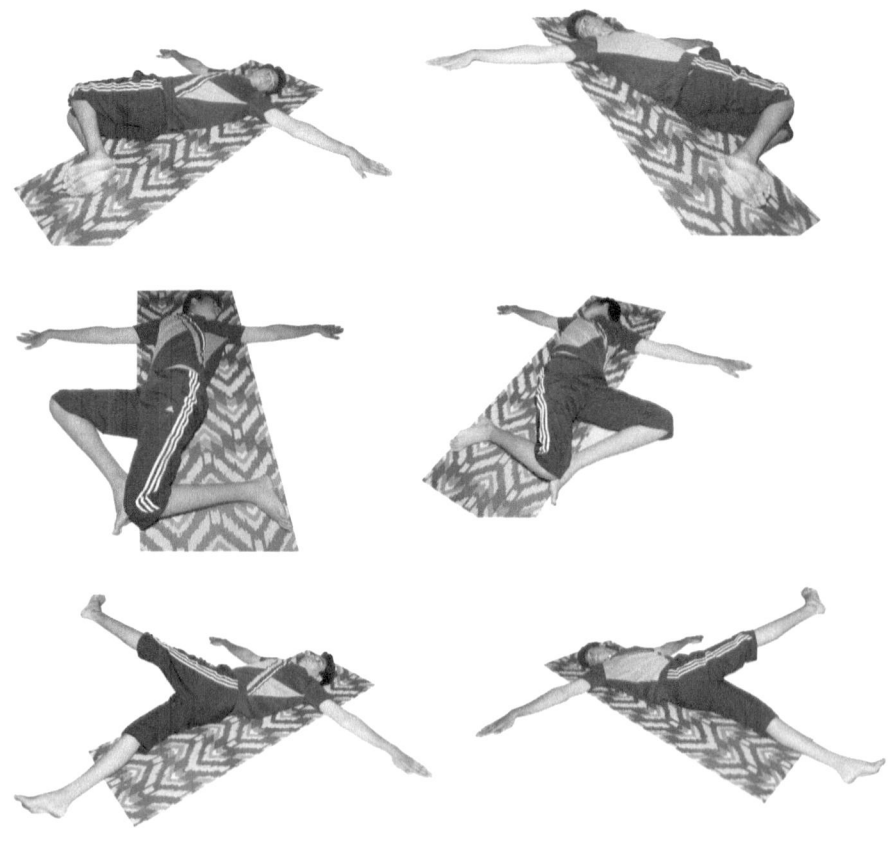

NATRAJA – DANCING LORD SHIVA; ASANA - POSE

Steps:

- ❖ Make yourself in Shava Asana pose. Spread your arms like wings at right angle to the body with palms touching the floor.
- ❖ Now bend your knees and drag your feet on the floor towards your hips. The soles of the feet should completely touch the ground.
- ❖ Now move both bent knees to the left until the left knee touches the ground, as a result the right knee will be lying on your left knee and right thigh on the left thigh. Simultaneously, turn the head to the right and look at your right palm.
- ❖ Move your head to the right and gaze at your right side keeping your shoulders straight touching the ground.
- ❖ After a while, move your head and paired knees and body back to centre in straight line.
- ❖ Now repeat all steps with bent knees towards right side and head left side, keeping rest of the body same.
- ❖ If someone faces problem of bending knees than this Asana can be done even without bending knees. In that case everything will remain same except that only one straight leg will move opposite to head direction as can be seen in pictures.

BENEFITS:

- ➤ It stretches and tones muscles like biceps and triceps.

PRECAUTIONS:

- ➤ It should be done under supervision of trained Yoga teacher.

5. SARVANGAASANA

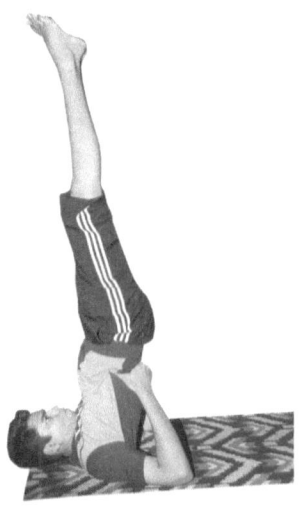

Sarvanga –All body parts; Asana – Pose

Steps:

- ❖ Make yourself in Shava Asana. Now raise whole body towards sky in such a way that that only shoulder and head is on the ground.
- ❖ While inverting yourself balance your raised body with the help of your hands holding the back with bent elbows on the the floor, making broad base for supporting upright straight body.

❖ Try to keep raised part of body straight as shown in picture.
❖ During this maintain normal breathing and stay in the posture for a while.
❖ Now slowly slowly bring down raised part of body on the floor.
❖ Remove your hands from holding back position to relaxed flat position as in Shava Asana.

BENEFITS:

➢ It smoothens the functioning of thyroid and parathyroid glands, brain, digestive system, venous system, excretory system and cardiac muscles.
➢ It provides flexibility to the spine.

PRECAUTIONS:

➢ This Asana is prevention not cure so any person suffering from Blood pressure problems, Glaucoma and Chronic thyroid must avoid it.
➢ Consult their physician before doing this Aasana.

6. NAUKA ASANA

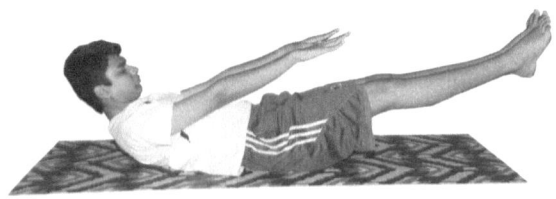

NAUKA = BOAT, ASANA = POSTURE OR POSE

Steps:

- ❖ Make yourself in Shava Asana pose.
- ❖ Now take a deep breath and raise your body in _/ wedge shape like boat as shown in picture.
- ❖ Take support of your stretched arms to lift your torso and feet simultaneously.
- ❖ In this pose the abdominal muscles contracts.
- ❖ Be in this pose as long as you feel you can comfortably tolerate.
- ❖ Maintain normal breathing and come back slowly to the ground and relax.

BENEFITS:

> It contracts abdominal muscles, stresses naval portion, stretches biceps and triceps.
> It is very effective in hernia problems.

PRECAUTIONS:

> Do not practice this yoga if you have blood pressure problems, headaches, asthama, cardiac problems, pregnancy, menstrual cycle or migraine.

7. SETUBANDH ASANA

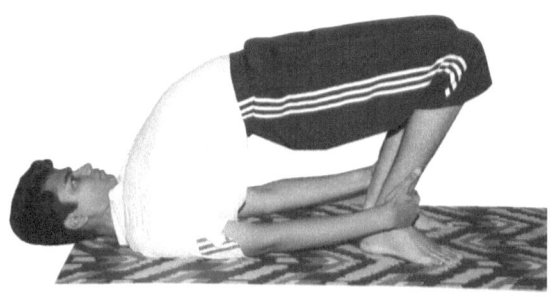

SETU – BRIDGE; BANDHA – BIND; ASANA – POSE

Steps:

- ❖ Make yourself in Shava Asana pose.
- ❖ Now bend your knees slowly and bring your feet just in straight line of knee.
- ❖ While breathing in, slowly raise your back away from the ground as shown in picture.
- ❖ While doing so hold your ankle with your hand giving a locked bridge structure.
- ❖ Maintain normal breathing.
- ❖ Hold the posture for a while and then come back slowly to Shava Asana pose.

BENEFITS:

> It relaxes the back muscles, nervous system, digestive system, respiratory system, menstrual cycle.
> It gives a good workout to the torso.
> It reduces thyroid problems, bone problems.

PRECAUTIONS:

> Do not practice this asana if you are suffering from spinal and neck problems.

8. MATSYA ASANA

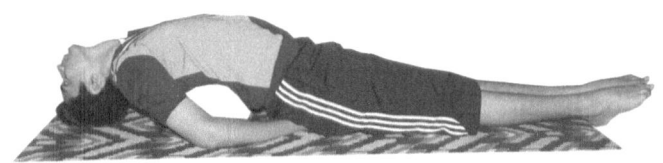

Matsya – Fish, Asana = Pose

Steps:

- ❖ Make yourself in Shava Asana pose.
- ❖ Now keep your hands underneath the hips, palms facing down.
- ❖ Breathe and slowly lift your chest pulling head upwards but well supported on the ground as shown in picture.

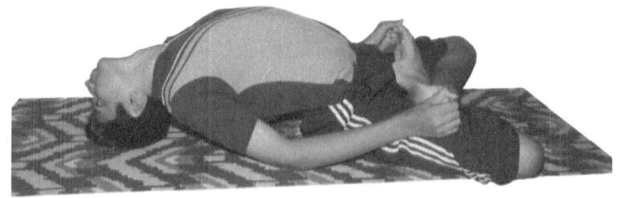

- ❖ This Asana can be done in other way also. Sit on the floor with folded legs as in Padma Asana. Hold your folded toe with your hands as shown in picture.

❖ Now bend upper torso backwards in arch shape till your head rests on the ground.

❖ Now hold this pose as per body's comfort tolerable limit. Breathe gently.

❖ Straighten up your head on the ground, bring the raised chest to flat position on the floor. Bring the hands back along the sides of the body. Relax.

BENEFITS:

➢ It helps in respiratory disorders, stretches the chest and neck and smoothens the functioning of glands.

➢ It relaxes the neck and shoulders.

PRECAUTIONS:

➢ Do not practice this Asana if you have blood pressure problems, migraine, insomnia or any back or neck problems.

9. PAWANMUKT ASANA

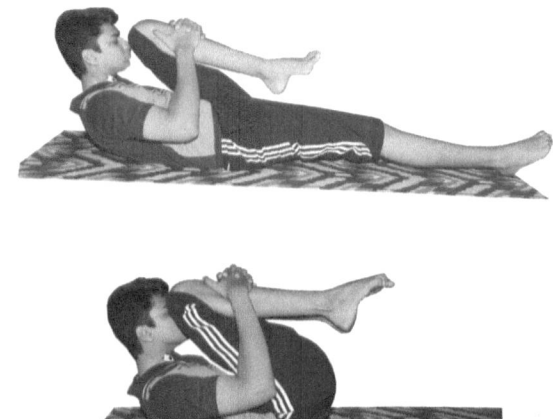

PAVANA = WIND, MUKTA = RELIEVE, ASANA = POSE

Steps:

- ❖ Make yourself in Shava Asana pose.
- ❖ Bend your right knee and pull it towards your face by holding bent knee with both hands till it touches your nose. For touching your nose lift your head also towards your bent knee as shown in picture. Stay in this pose for a while and then unbent your knee and relax it straight and so is your head also on the floor.
- ❖ Now repeat the same with left knee also.

❖ Now repeat the same with both knees together.
❖ During breathing when you breathe out hold the knee tightly but when you breathe in relax your knee holding.

BENEFITS:

➢ As the name suggests it allows gastric gas to pass conveniently.
➢ It strengthens muscular system, digestive system, circulation of blood in hip joints.

PRECAUTIONS:

➢ Do not practice this Asana if one is suffering from acidity, hernia, cardiac problem, menstrual problems, blood pressure problems, spinal or neck problems.

10. HALA ASANA

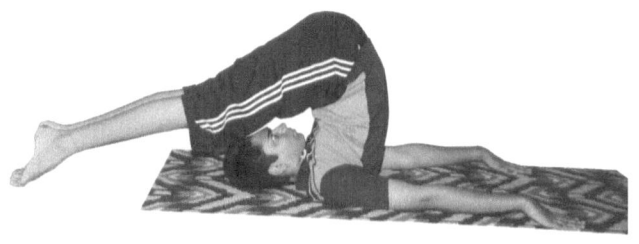

HALA = PLOW, ASANA – POSE, POSTURE

Steps:

- ❖ Make yourself in Shava Asana pose.
- ❖ During inhaling with the help of abdominal muscles and raise your legs straight upwards facing sky.
- ❖ Now hold hips and back with your hands and raise them away from the ground slowly.
- ❖ It will provide ease to legs to move back crossing over your head till they touches ground as shown in the picture.
- ❖ Ensure your body's comfort zone.
- ❖ Stay in this pose as per your body's comfort limit.
- ❖ Now while exhaling slowly bring your legs in reverse direction till heels touch the ground.

BENEFITS:

> ➢ It helps in relaxing of nervous system, menopause, gives flexibility to muscles.
> ➢ It smoothens thyroid gland functioning and improves immunity.
> ➢ It rejuvenates body and mind.

PRECAUTIONS:

> ➢ Do not practice this Asana if one is pregnant or suffering from menstrual problems, blood pressure problems, spinal or neck problems.

11. VISHNU ASANA

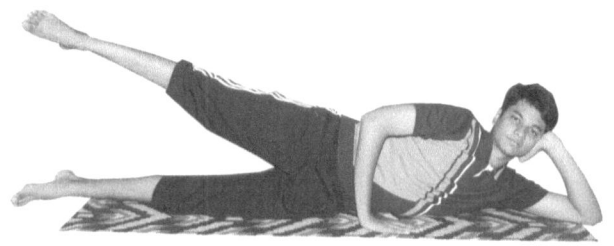

VISHNU =INDIAN GOD (THE PRESERVER), ASANA – POSE, POSTURE

Instructions:

❖ Relax and make yourself in Shava Asana. Now move your body at 90 degree to floor in such a way that only one side of your body touches the ground as shown in picture.

❖ If you moved towards right side of your body then take out your right hand and support your head with firm elbow footing on the floor as shown in the picture.

❖ Now bring left hand palm on the floor just in close proximity of chest as shown in picture.

❖ Keep your legs straight, one above another parallelly placed. Now raise your left leg upwards as much as it can go up and then slowly bring it down by rotating clockwise and then going in other direction continuing clockwise circular motion.

❖ After 3-4 circular movements bring down leg in resting position.

❖ Now lie on your back and repeat all steps with other side of your body.

BENEFITS:

➢ It helps in strengthening your lower body especially the pelvic joint through circular movements.

➢ It brings flexibility.

PRECAUTIONS:

➢ Do not practice this Asana if one has undergone through any abdominal or pelvic surgery.

12. KATICHAKRA ASANA

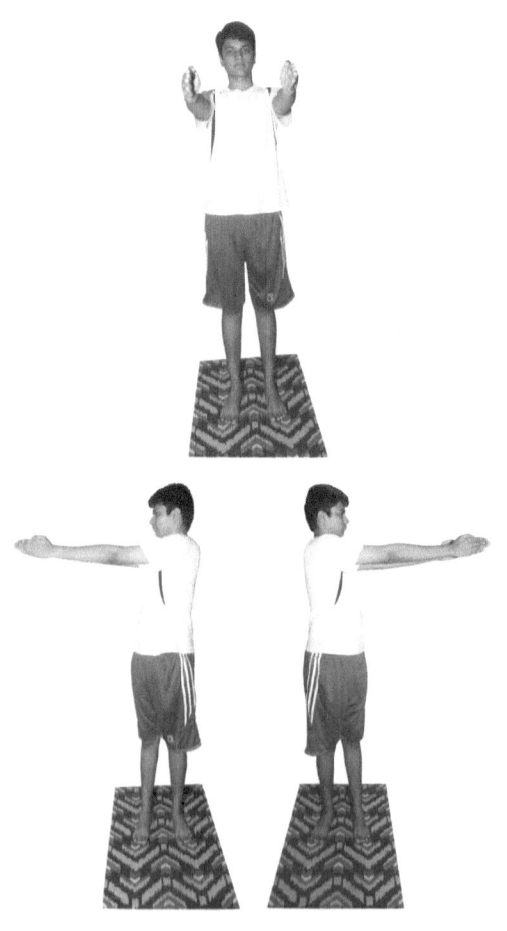

KATI=WAIST, CHAKRA =WHEEL, ASANA – POSE, POSTURE

Steps:

❖ Join your feet together and stand in attentive pose.

❖ Now take your hands together, parallel to each other upto your chest level as shown in the picture.

❖ While breathing out rotate your waist towards the right direction and try to look backwards as much as possible by rotating your head also towards right direction over the right shoulder as shown in the picture.

❖ Now inhale and return to the centre pose.

❖ Now exhale and repeat the yoga posture with your left side as shown in picture.

❖ In the end bring down hands in relaxed mode.

BENEFITS:

➤ It warms up and offers flexibility to muscles, neck, shoulder, spine and waist and keeps constipation at bay.

PRECAUTIONS:

➤ Avoid during pregnancy, spinal disorder, hernia, slip disc or any abdominal surgery.

➤ Avoid jerk during body movements.

➤ Co-ordinate movements with breathing patterns.

13. HASTAPADA ASANA

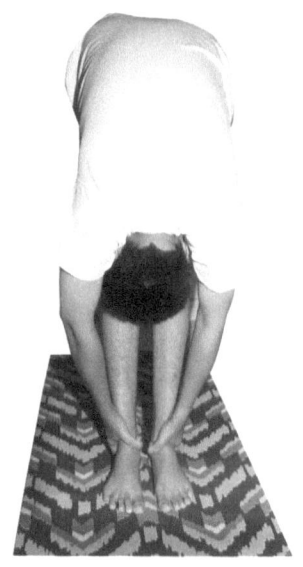

HASTA- HAND; PADAH- FOOT; ASANA – POSE, POSTURE

Steps:

- ❖ Relax, join your feet side to side and stand straight straight in attentive pose.
- ❖ Keep your arms down on both sides. Stretch your arms upwards, parallel to each other, touching each ear and breathe in.

❖ Now while breathing out bend upper body above hips towards forward, keeping your head in between arms without bending spine and finally bring down towards the feet in such a way that nose rests in between knees and palm should touch ground as shown in the picture..

❖ Stay in this pose as long as your body's comfort zone allows.

❖ Inhale and release your arms and come back in original standing position with arms down in the similar way as we moved from standing position.

BENEFITS:

➢ Since it involve deep bending from abdominal portion so it abdominal organs, stretches back muscles.

➢ It increases blood supply to the nervous system.

PRECAUTIONS:

➢ Since it involves back U bending so people suffering from any back and abdominal problems should avoid it.

14. ARDH CHAKRASANA

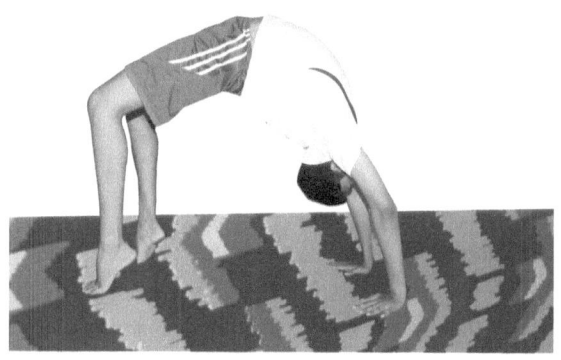

ARDHA= HALF; CHAKRA= WHEEL; ASANA – POSE, POSTURE

Steps:

- ❖ Relax, join your feet side to side and stand straight with shoulder width distance in between them.
- ❖ Keep your arms down on both sides. Stretch your arms upwards, parallel to each other, touching each ear and breathe in.
- ❖ Now push your upper body above waist, backwards till your hands (palm) touches the ground as shown in picture.
- ❖ Hold for a while, slowly inhale and return anticlockwise to your original position.

BENEFITS:

> ➤ It stretches the whole body (abdominal, chest. shoulder, pelvis and thighs).

PRECAUTIONS:

> ➤ This asana should be avoided in pregnancy, hip or back problems, ulcer, hernia, brain problems or any blood pressure problems.

15. VEERABHADRA ASANA

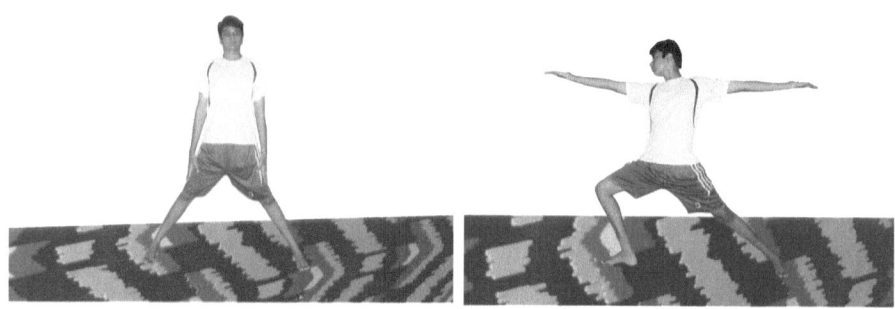

VEERA - CHIVALEROUS,; BHADRA - GOOD; ASANA – POSE

Steps:

- ❖ Stand upright with your legs wide apart with arms stretched parallel to ground on your sides
- ❖ Move your left foot facing left side of you.
- ❖ The other foot will turn inward to make a 45 Degree angle.
- ❖ Twist your body to left completely.
- ❖ Go forward on your left knee making a 90 Degree angle; make sure that your knee doesn't cross over the toe as shown in picture.
- ❖ Let the other leg stretch properly
- ❖ Hold for 10 seconds and repeat on the other side.

BENEFITS:

> It rejuvenates shoulders, arms, legs and lower back and revives stamina.
> It enhances body balance.

PRECAUTIONS:

> Avoid this posture if you are suffering from spinal orders, blood pressure problems, arthritis or diarrhea.

16. TRIKON ASANA

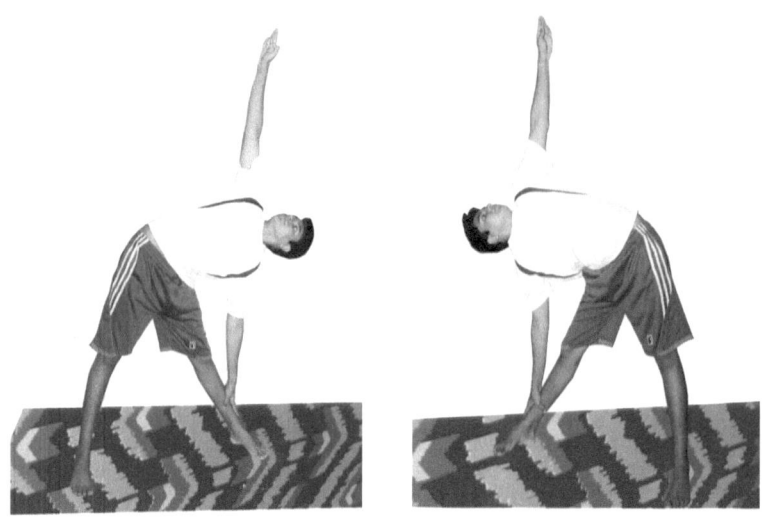

TRIKON – TRIANGLE: ASANA – POSE

Instructions:

❖ Stand upright with your legs wide apart with arms stretched to your side parallel to ground.

❖ Your arms should be in sleeping straight line with open stretched palms.

❖ Now bend from your hip towards right along with set of straight hands without disturbing straight line of hands till finger of right hand touches floor or ankle (whatever is convenient to you), making perpendicular to the ground as shown in picture.

❖ Stay for a while in this pose and then come back to original straight upright position with hands parallel to ground.

❖ Now repeat with bending hip towards left side as shown in picture.

BENEFITS:

➤ It stretches and strengthens the thighs, hips, groins, calves, shoulders, chest, spine, soothes nervous system, knees, and ankles

➤ It improves appetite, digestion, blood circulation, flatulence and posture

➤ It helps in relieving acidity, flat feet, neck pain, osteoporosis and sciatica

PRECAUTIONS:

➤ People with lower back problems, neck problems, diarrhoea, headache and blood pressure problems should avoid it.

17. VRIKSHASA ASANA

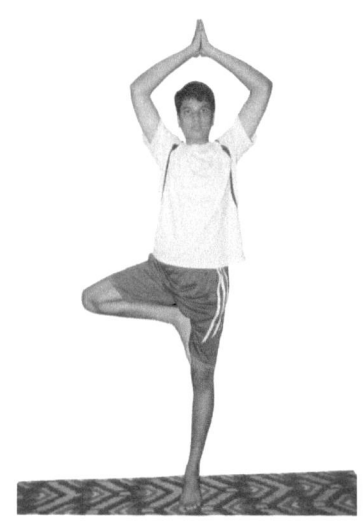

VRIKSHA - TREE; ASANA – POSE

Instructions:

- ❖ Stand erect in attentive pose with the feet together and the arms by your sides
- ❖ Bend the right leg at the knee, raise the lower part of right leg to the right thigh and bring the sole of the right foot as high up the inside of the left thigh as possible.
- ❖ Now balancing whole body weight on the left foot, lift both arms over the head keeping the elbows unbent and joining

the palms together as shown in picture. Hold the posture for a while.

❖ Now bring down arms and right leg. After relaxing a bit repeat steps on the other leg.

BENEFITS:

➢ This pose rejuvenates and stretches the legs, back and arms, and invigorates you.

➢ It improves focus, concentration and brings balance and equilibrium to your mind..

➢ It helps those who are suffering from sciatica.

PRECAUTIONS:

➢ Avoid doing this posture if you are suffering from migraine, insomnia or blood pressure problems.

18. UTKATASANA

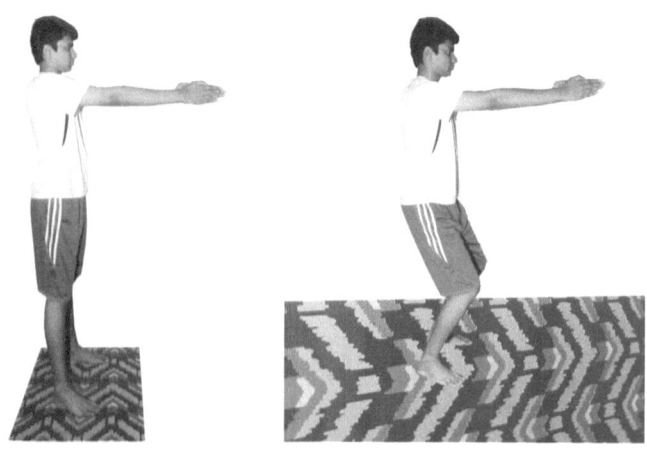

UTKAT=INTENSE; ASANA= POSE

Instructions:

- ❖ Relax and stand straight with shoulder width distance between your feet
- ❖ Now bring your straight hands to the front with open palms.
- ❖ Make sure that elbow should be in straight alignment with arm as shown in picture.
- ❖ Now try to pull down your whole body towards the ground by little bending of knees (from 180 degree to some 120 degree angle) as shown in picture.

❖ During the whole process keep your hands steady parallel to the ground.
❖ Hold your body for a while and then come back to original position by lifting your body upwards with knees making straight line 180 degree angle.
❖ Bring down your hands in relaxed pose.

BENEFITS:

➢ It tones the back and lower part of body (from hip downwards to toe) and chest muscles.
➢ It enhances body balance of the body, concentration and focus.

PRECAUTIONS:

➢ Avoid this pose if you are suffering from insomnia, knee pain, arthritis, headache, sprained ankle or injured ligaments.

19. JANUSHIRASANA

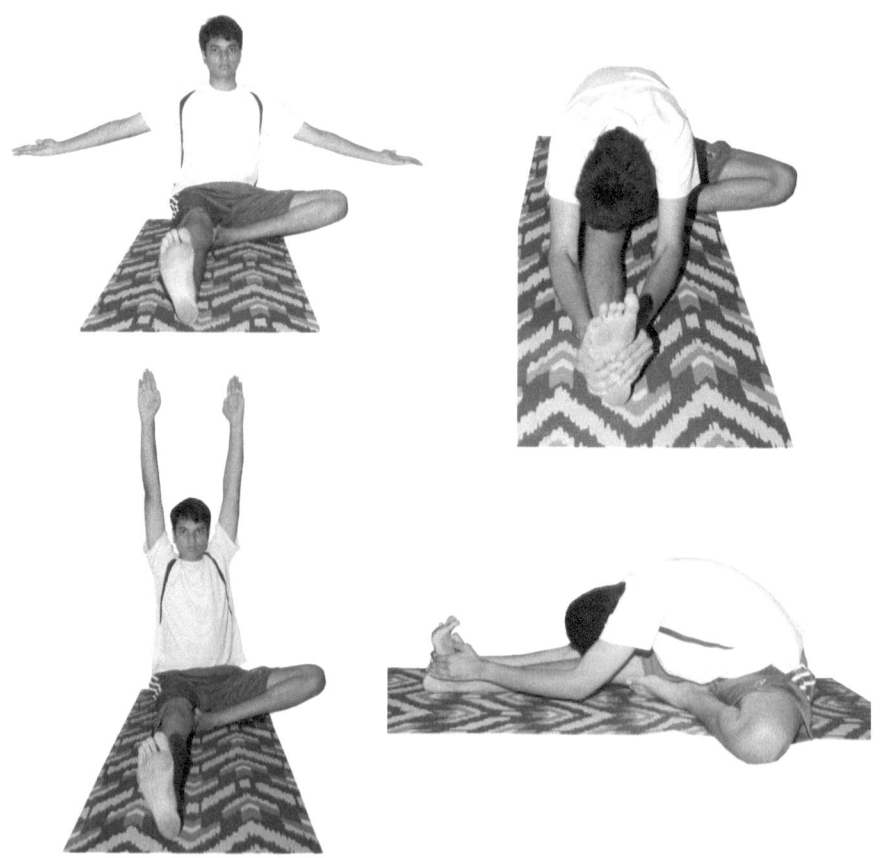

JANUSHIRA= HEAD TO KNEE POSE; ASANA= POSE

Steps:

- ❖ Sit down on the mat. Spread your legs out straight in front of you. Make sure that upper part of body above waist should be straight upright.
- ❖ Now bend the one of the knee and bring that foot against the thigh of other foot. Make sure bent knee should maintain its touch on the floor as shown in the picture.
- ❖ Now inhale and slowly lift both side arms straight upwards. Rotate your waist little towards the stretched foot.
- ❖ Along with exhaling bend whole upward straight body (above the waist) forward till your chin touches the toe of extended straight foot as shown in picture.
- ❖ Stay in this pose as long as your body comfortably allows you. Keep breathing.
- ❖ Finally return to original position by reverse movements.
- ❖ Repeat all steps with the other side so that body stretches in balanced manner.

BENEFITS:

- ➤ It strengthens lower back, shoulders and abdominal organs.

PRECAUTIONS:

- ➤ Avoid this yoga posture if you are suffering from chronic back pain, knee pain, arthritis, headache or insomnia.
- ➤ Take special care and proceed gently with this yoga posture under supervision and guidance of trained yoga teacher.

20. PASCHIMOTTANA ASANA

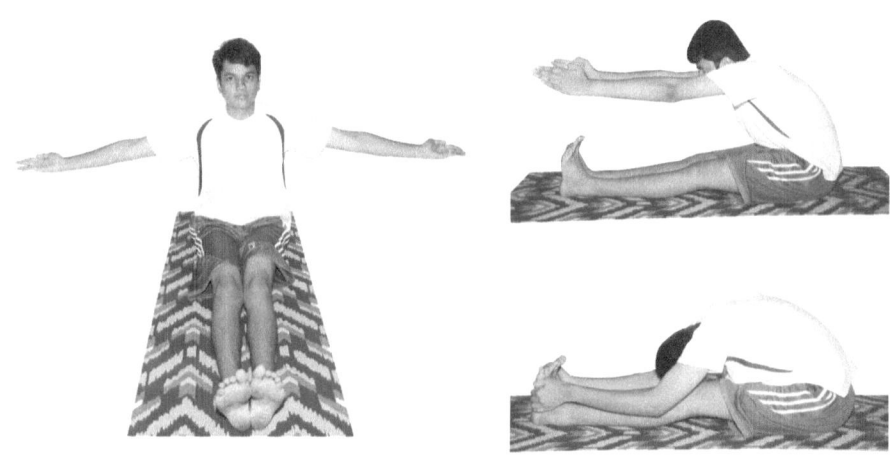

PASCHIM = WEST; UTTANA = STRETCHED OUT; ASANA= POSE

Steps:

- ❖ Sit down with the spreaded straight legs in front of you with straight upright torso
- ❖ Now lift both arms straight upwards, parallel to each other.
- ❖ Now bend from hip your upright straight body forward till your hand fingers touches or holds foot toe as shown in picture.
- ❖ Relax and breathe deeply for a while.

❖ While inhaling with the help of your arms, come back up to the sitting relaxed position.

BENEFITS:

➢ It strengthens and stretches shoulder, abdominal and pelvic organs.

PRECAUTIONS:

➢ Avoid this yoga posture if you are suffering from back pain, knee pain, arthritis, headache or insomnia.

21. POORVOTTANA ASANA

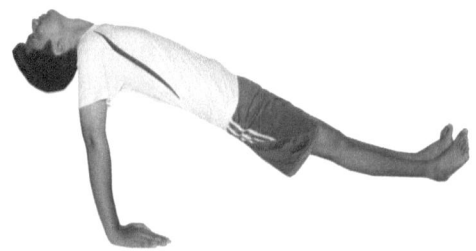

Poorva = east; uttana = stretch; asana = Pose

Instructions:

- ➤ This is famously known as Upper Plank Pose.
- ➤ Sit down on the floor with spreaded straight feet on the ground. Join your feet side by side.
- ➤ Put your side arms on the floor with palm lying flat on the ground with fingers pointing towards toe.
- ➤ While inhaling lift up hips, pushing whole body upwards keeping your heels mounted on the floor.
- ➤ During lifting make sure body should be in straight line like a plank, balanced by flat palms of unbent straight hands on the floor as can be seen in the picture.
- ➤ Allow your head leisurely hanging towards the ground.

> Stay in the pose as long as you feel comfortable and then bring down hip along with whole body slowly to flat position on the ground.

BENEFITS:

> It increases the strength and stamina of thigh, back, wrist and shoulders (including joints).

PRECAUTIONS:

> If you are overweight, raise your body only few inches, and stay only few seconds in final position.
> Wrist and neck problems people should avoid this Asana.

22. *ARDH MATSYENDRA ASANA*

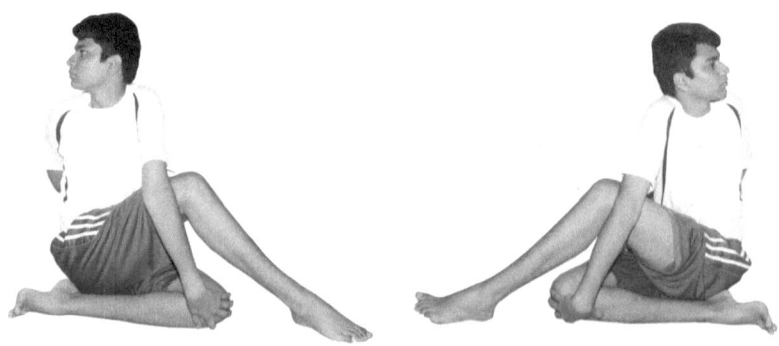

A̲ʀᴅʜᴀ = ʜᴀʟꜰ; ᴍᴀᴛꜱʏᴀ = ꜰɪꜱʜ; ɪɴᴅʀᴀ = ʀᴜʟᴇʀ (I̲ɴᴅɪᴀɴ ᴍʏᴛʜᴏʟᴏɢɪᴄᴀʟ ɢᴏᴅ)

Steps:

- ❖ Sit down erect on the ground with the straight legs spreaded in front of you with joined feet side by side.
- ❖ Now bend the left knee inwards and place the heel of the left foot underside the right hip.
- ❖ Now move the right leg over the left knee and rest your right foot just adjacent to left knee as shown in pictures.
- ❖ Rest your left hand on the right knee and the right hand behind away from you balancing body alongwith rotating shoulder and face in the direction of right hand as seen in pictures.
- ❖ Keep your torso upright straight as can be seen in the pictures.

❖ Stay in this pose with relaxed breathing as long as body allows.

❖ Now release all parts of the body to their relaxed pose.

❖ Repeat all steps with the other side.

BENEFITS:

➢ It offers flexibility to spine.

➢ It stretches chest and enhances oxygen supply to the lungs

PRECAUTIONS:

➢ Do not force your body beyond comfort zone.

➢ Do under the supervision and guidance of trained yoga teacher.

23. BADHAKON ASANA

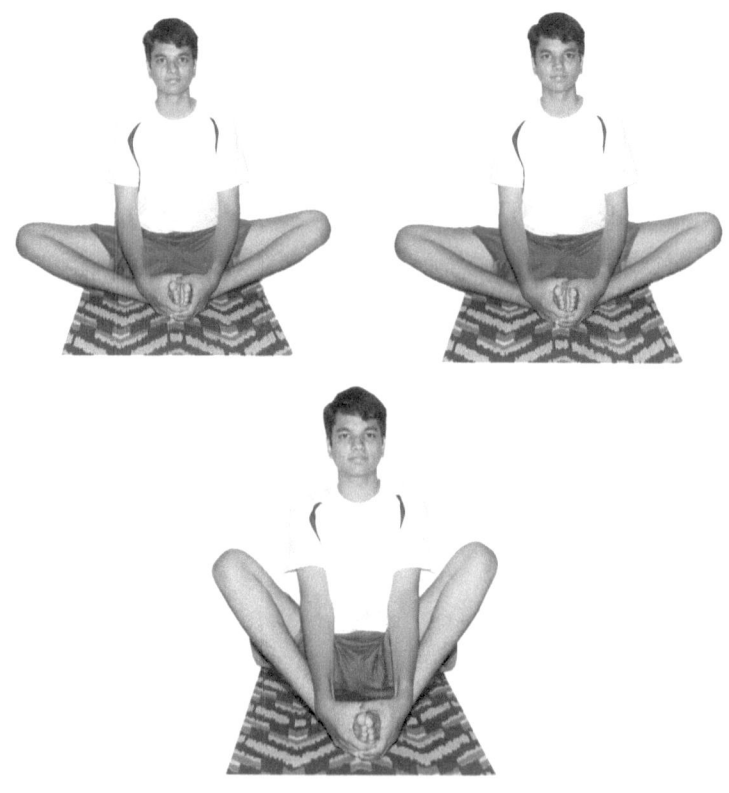

BADHA = BARRIER, KONA = ANGLE, ASANA = POSE

Steps:

* This Asana can be called butterfly jogging except that you will jog only on ground while butterfly jogs in the air.
* Sit down with straight upper body and spread straight legs out in front of you.
* Make your side feet parallel to the ground and now bring your feet inwards towards the pelvis in such a way that soles of both feet lock together like feet salutation.
* Now hold your both locked feets in your both hands in interlocked position.
* Try to pull heels of locked feet inwards as much as possible as shown in picture.
* Now while inhaling push down thighs and knees towards the ground gently as can be seen in picture.
* Now assume both bent legs as wings of butterfly and flap them up and down. In the beginning flap slowly as one start learning to fly and gradually pick up speed as expert butterfly with normal breathing.
* You will feel the apparent deep stretching in the inner thighs.
* Maintain posture of upright body erect.
* In the end relax the legs by spreading them out in front of you.

BENEFITS:

➢ It gives stretching and flexibility to the inner thighs, hips and knees.
➢ It facilitates relaxation from long sedentary state of body and eases bowel movement and menstrual cycle.

PRECAUTIONS:

➢ Avoid if you have knee problem, lower back disorder or sciatica.
➢ Do not perform this pose without sitting cushion support.

24. MARJARIASAN

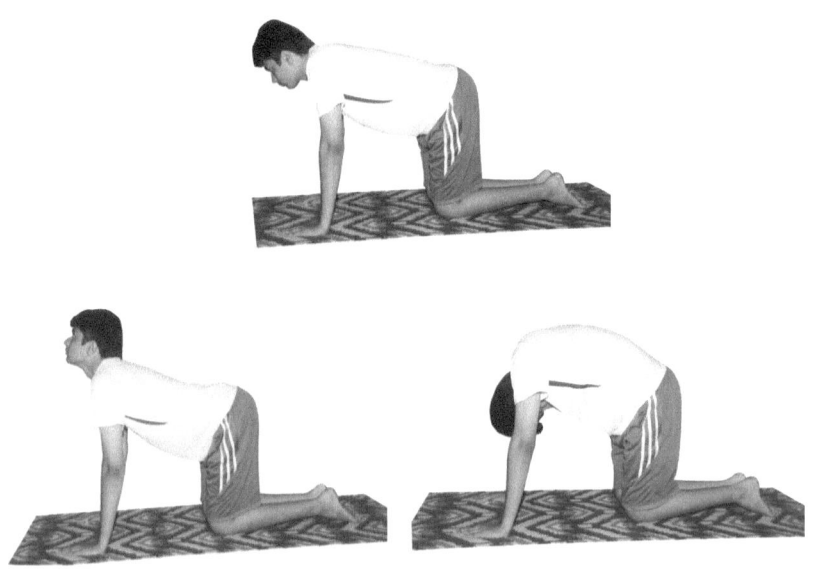

MARJARI = CAT; ASANA= POSE

Steps:

❖ Relax and bring down your both forlimbs(hands) and hindlimbs(L shape bent feet) on the ground such a way that whole body weight is balanced on both palms and soles of feet placed on the ground like cat stands as shown in picture.

❖ Your arms should be straight in line with the shoulders

* Keep your knees comfortably wide apart.
* Keep your head like cat looking forward as seen in picture.
* While breathing in lift your head as cat looks you when cat and you stand facing each other as shown in picture.
* Stay in the pose with deep breathing.
* While exhaling drop down your head and bend your back making reverse U, as shown in picture.
* Stay in this pose as long as body allows then return to human standing pose.

BENEFITS:

➤ It makes spine flexible and increases strength of wrist and shoulder joints.
➤ It facilitates smooth functioning of circulatory system, nervous system and digestive system.

PRECAUTIONS:

➤ Avoid this Asana if you have wrist, shoulder, back or neck problems.

25. SHISHU ASANA

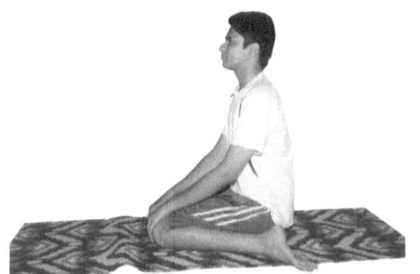 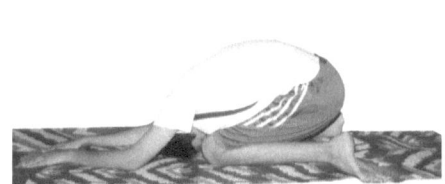

Sʜɪsʜᴜ=ʙᴀʙʏ; Asᴀɴᴀ= Pᴏsᴇ

Steps:

- ❖ Sit down like a toddler sits on his heels.
- ❖ While sitting on the heels, raise your both hands straight upwards parallel to each other and bend your whole upper body (including hands) forward till your forehead and palms of straight hands touches the floor as can be seen in the picture.
- ❖ Slowly push down your chest against the thighs.
- ❖ Stay for a while.
- ❖ Now slowly lift your upper body to normal position and relax.

BENEFITS:

> ➢ It relaxes and rejuvenates the back muscles and nervous system..
> ➢ It eases bowl movement.

PRECAUTIONS:

> ➢ Avoid this pose if you are suffering from diarrhoea, back or knee injuries or pregnant.

26. CHAKKI CHALANA ASASNA

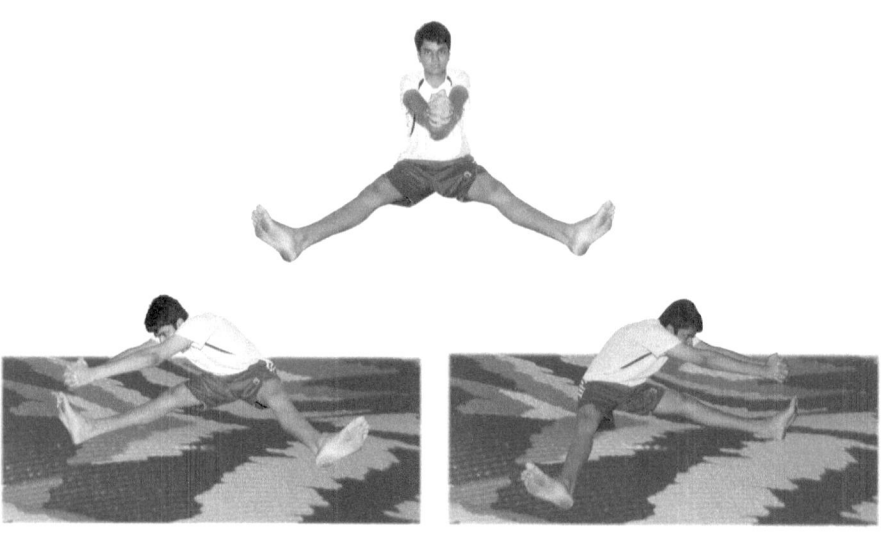

CHAKKI = GRINDER, CHALANA = TO ROTATE; ASANA= POSE

Steps:

- ❖ Sit down and spread your leg in V shape with maximum distance between your feet. Interlock both your hands as your are holding something very tightly as seen in the picture and spread out in horizontal sleeping line with shoulder in front of you.
- ❖ Now start rotating upper part of body including spreaded hands from the waist like making a circle from compass.

❖ Pace of rotation should be adjusted in such a way that when body comes forward you should breathe in while breathe out as it approaches backward.

❖ Try to keep legs undisturbed as can be seen in the picture.

BENEFITS:

➢ A good preventive for sciatica

➢ It stretches chest, groin, back, abs and arm muscles

➢ It helps in shedding any type of extra belly fat and prevention for sciatica.

PRECAUTIONS:

➢ Avoid if you are suffering from blood pressure problem, slip disc, headaches, hernia, abdominal surgery.

27. DHANURA ASANA

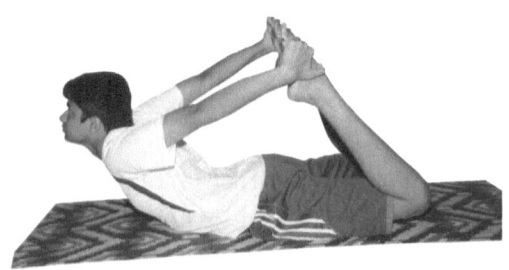

DHANURA = BOW; ASANA= POSE

Steps:

❖ Relax and lie down facing floor with wide spread feet and straight arms resting on your sides.
❖ Now bend your knees and lift lower part of leg.
❖ Now raise your hands and get hold of ankles of lifted leg.
❖ Pull your legs and simultaneously raise your torso also as can be seen in the picture.
❖ You should look forward in joyous mood.
❖ Stay in the pose as long as body allows.
❖ Finally breathe out and release all body parts in relaxed mode.

BENEFITS:

> ➤ It gives good stretching to all body parts, eases bowl movement, make spine flexible.
> ➤ It relaxes whole body.

PRECAUTIONS:

> ➤ Avoid this pose in pregnancy and if you are suffering from blood pressure problem, slip disc, headaches, hernia, abdominal surgery.

28. BHUJANG ASANA

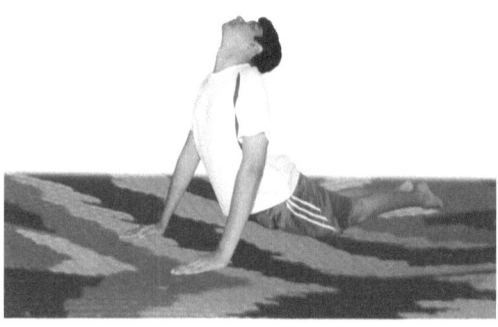

BHUJANG = SNAKE (COBRA); ASANA= POSE

Steps:

- ❖ Lie down on the floor in such a way that your face, abdomen, knee and toes should touch the floor surface.
- ❖ While inhaling lift your chest upwards and slowly make hand straight standing on ground on palms.
- ❖ Both feet should be fully stretched straight and close to each other.
- ❖ Lower part of body till naval should touch the ground.
- ❖ But eyes should be focussed upwards towards sky as shown in picture.

BENEFITS:

> It stretches and strengthens back, chest, shoulders and neck.
> It relaxes and tones whole body.
> It helps in asthma and smoothes blood circulation.

PRECAUTIONS:

> Avoid this Asana in pregnancy, asthmatic attack, spinal problems or operated for hernia.

29. VIPARITA SHALABHASANA

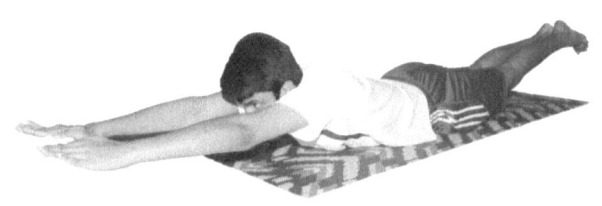

VIPARITA = INVERTED; SHALABH = LOCUST; Asana= Pose

Steps:

- ❖ Lie down inverted straight on the floor in such a way that your abdomen, knees, nose and finger toes should face floor.
- ❖ Now we will streamline our body by bringing straight legs close together.
- ❖ Now spread out your straight arms in front of your eyes.
- ❖ Now inhale and lift all your body up as you want to fly upwards as can be seen in the picture.
- ❖ Stay in the pose as long as your body wants and then breathe out and lower down all raised part of body which were engaged in effort of flying.

BENEFITS:

> It stretches and strengthens back, chest, shoulders and neck.
> It relaxes and tones whole body.
> It smoothes blood circulation

PRECAUTIONS:

> Avoid this Asana in pregnancy and any abdominal surgery.

30. SHALABHASANA

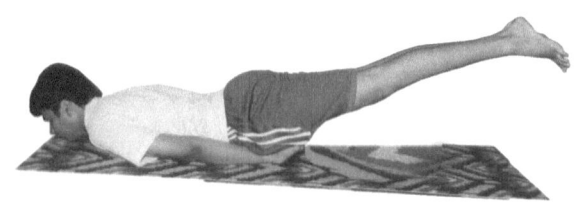

SHALABH = LOCUST; ASANA= POSTURE/POSE

Steps:

- ❖ Lie down inverted straight on the floor in such a way that your abdomen, knees, nose and finger toes should face floor.
- ❖ Lift the both straight legs up with the support of straight hands and palms on the floor as shown in the picture.
- ❖ Stay in the pose as long as you can.
- ❖ While exhaling bring down both legs slowly.

BENEFITS:

> ➤ It stretches and strengthens the nerves and muscles of arms, back, neck and shoulders
> ➤ It revitalize abdominal organs and helps digestion.

PRECAUTIONS:

> ➤ Avoid this Asana in pregnancy and any abdominal injury.

31. PADMA ASANA

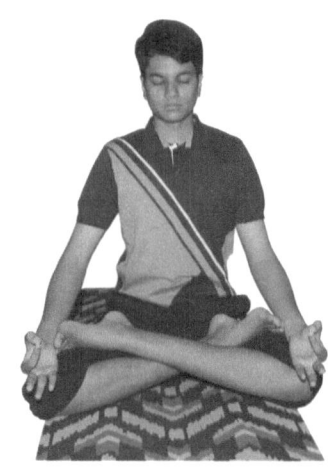

PADMA = LOTUS; ASANA= POSE

Steps:

- ❖ Sit down straight on the floor, with legs stretched out in front of you with erect spine.
- ❖ Now bend your right knee sideways and fold leg and bring right foot closer to you.
- ❖ Place your right heel on the left thigh.
- ❖ Similarly fold your left leg and bring it closer to you.
- ❖ Place the left heel on your right thigh as can be seen in the picture.

❖ Rest palms of both hands on their respective knees facing sky.
❖ Now took your hand thumb and touch index finger making sign of O other fingers will be in stretched out pose as shown in the picture.

BENEFITS:

➢ It is the most ideal sitting correct posture.
➢ It increases focus and concentration.
➢ It calms down restlessness and anxiety of the brain..
➢ It helps in restoring vitality of whole body.
➢ It improves apetite.
➢ Meditation and Pranayam is done only in this pose for maximum benefits.
➢ It is an excellent stretching workout for knees.

PRECAUTIONS:

➢ Avoid this pose if you are suffering from ankle injury, sprain in leg, back pain or have undergone a recent knee surgery.

32. GOMUKHA ASANA

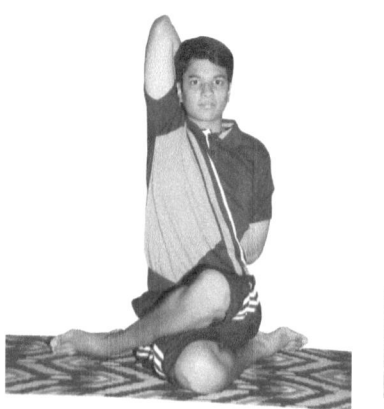 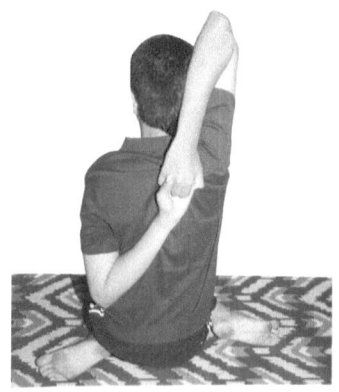

Go=cow, mukh = mouth; Asana= Posture/Pose

Steps:

❖ Sit down straight with erect upper part of the body.
❖ Spread straight legs out in front of you.
❖ Now bend the left leg and put the left foot on the ground over the right knee.
❖ Now Bend the right leg and fold it so that it is resting on the ground with the right heel near the left hip.
❖ Adjust the right knee so that it rests on the left knee.
❖ Place the hands either on the knee or on the respective foot whichever is comfortable.

❖ Hold the head, back and neck straight as shown in the picture. Close the eyes and relax.
❖ To release the asana, release the hands to your sides. Straighten the bottom leg in front of you. Straighten the other leg returning to sitting position.
❖ Now practice with the other side.

BENEFITS:

➢ It gives good stretching to hips, thighs, ankles and chest and shoulders.

PRECAUTIONS:

➢ Avoid this Asana in case of neck, knee, hip and shoulders injury.
➢ Do under the supervision and guidance of expert trained yoga teacher.

33. VAJRA ASANA

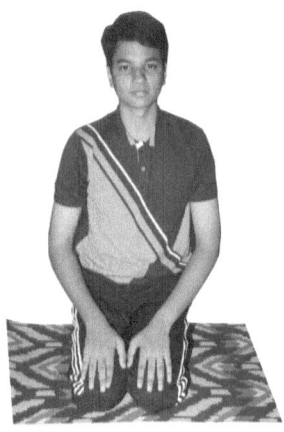

VAJRA=WAR WEAPON(THUNDERBOLT) USED BY INDIAN
MYTHOLOGICAL GOD(INDRA); ASANA= POSE

Steps:

- ❖ Relax and sit down on the floor.
- ❖ Bend your knees and fold your legs and sit in such a manner such that you sit on the heels.
- ❖ Place your hands on your lap exactly as shown in the picture.
- ❖ Stay in this pose pose for a while. One may feel pain in your feet or thighs if you are beginner. You can relax out your legs and can redo.
- ❖ Best time to do Vajrasana is just after meal.

BENEFITS:

> It relieves from Gastric problems, arthritis and sciatica.
> It helps in shedding extra fat from the hip region.
> It is the only posture which you can do immediately after the food.
> It helps in digestion.

PRECAUTIONS:

> Avoid this pose If you have had some leg injury.
> Please do this asana under supervision and expert guidance of expert yoga teacher.

34.   *SUPTVAJRA ASANA*

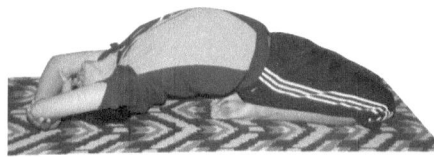 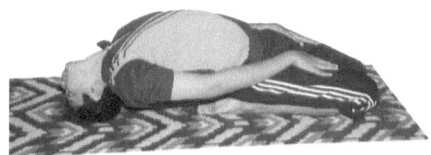

SUPTVAJRA=WAR WEAPON(SLEEPING/HORIZONTAL THUNDERBOT)
USED BY INDIAN GOD(INDRA); ASANA= POSE

Steps:

- ❖ Sit comfortably in Vajrasana.
- ❖ Keep your palms on the floor beside the hips with your fingers pointing to the front.
- ❖ Slowly bend back, putting the forearm and the elbow on the bottom to the left.
- ❖ Slowly bring down your head to the ground while arching the back. Place your hands on your thighs as shown in the picture..
- ❖ While inhaling with the support of the elbows and arms lift the chest higher keeping head on the floor.

❖ Now bend elbows and fold arms in such away that palm holding elbow of other hand.

❖ Take folded hands beyond your head and rests them on the floor like head as shown in the picture.

❖ Stay in this pose as long as body allows.

❖ Slowly return to the starting position by reversing all steps.

BENEFITS:

➢ It soothes spinal nerves and sciatic nerves.

➢ It gives good stretching to upper parts of the body, thighs and legs.

➢ It smoothes the functioning of digestive system, respiratory system and adrenal gland.

➢ It calms and relaxes mind.

PRECAUTIONS:

➢ Avoid this asana if you are pregnant or having blood pressure problems, slip disc, knee injury/surgery or in menstrual cycle.

35. *KUKKUTA ASANA*

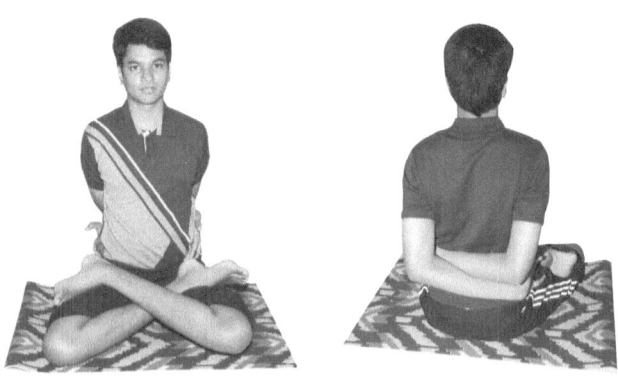

KUKKUTA=COCK. ROOSTER; ASANA= POSTURE/POSE

Steps:

* ❖ Sit down in the Lotus Pose (Padmasana).
* ❖ Put your arms in-between the gaps of your thighs and calf muscles, and your palms should touch the ground or floor through this gap.
* ❖ Now spread out your fingers, pointing forward.
* ❖ Push your palms on the floor as much as possible. Now start lifting your body, while inhaling as shown in the picture.
* ❖ Stay in this pose for a while.
* ❖ Exhale and and release the pose and get back to the ground.

BENEFITS:

> ➢ It stretches and strengthens arms, spine, shoulders, elbows and wrists.
> ➢ It increases concentration level and smoothes the functioning of the digestive system.

PRECAUTIONS:

> ➢ Avoid this asana If you have had any leg injury, back or spinal injury or pain.

36. BHADRA ASANA/ SUKHASANA

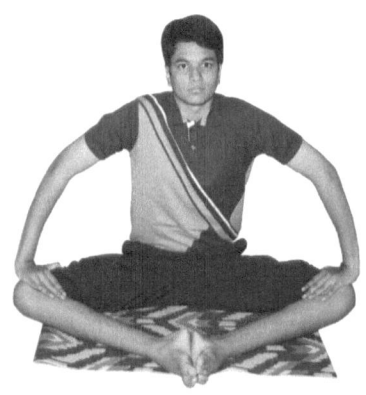

BHADRA=BENEFICIAL; ASANA= POSE

Instructions:

- ❖ Sit down with erect upper body.
- ❖ Spread out straight legs in front of you.
- ❖ Bend knees sideway and fold your legs simultaneously till soles of your feet touch each other.
- ❖ Now bend elbows also sideway and bring your hand towards your knee and rests your palm on the knees.
- ❖ Pull joined soles towards you as much as you can.
- ❖ Press down knees gently with rested palms as shown in picture.

❖ Knees shold be pressed down within body's comfort zone.
❖ Stay in the pose for a while and then relese the pose and return to starting relaxed pose.

BENEFITS:

➢ It relieves stiffness of leg joints
➢ It smoothes the functioning of excretory system organs.

PRECAUTIONS:

➢ If you have had some leg injury, please do not do this without expert guidance

37. MANDUK ASANA/ BHEKASANA

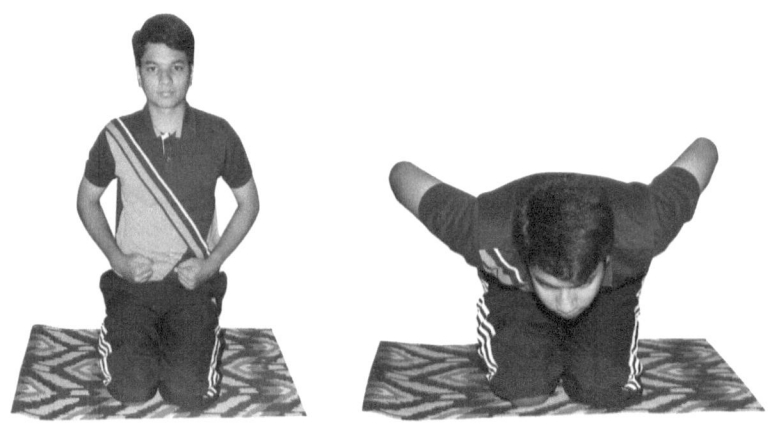

MANDUK=FROG; ASANA= POSTURE/POSE

Steps: *There are two ways to do this asana:*

WAY 1:

- Sit in Vajrasana.
- Now, make fists where thumbs should be inside.
- Put the fists at the naval region.
- Inhale deeply.
- With exhale bend forward and put maximum pressure on the naval area.

- While bending forward, your chest should touch your thigh and see ahead with open eyes just like as frog as shown in the picture.
- Maintain the pose as long as you can do.
- Inhale-exhale slowing while maintaining the pose.
- Come to Vajrasana with deep inhale.
- Perform it 3 to 5 times.

WAY 2:

- Sit in Vajrasana
- Put your left palm on your navel area and the right palm over the left palm.
- Inhale deeply.
- Exhale and bend forward and take suitable stretch on your naval region through your palms as shown in the picture.
- Hold the pose as long as you can with slow inhaling and exhaling.
- Come to Vajrasana with deep inhale.

BENEFITS:

- ➢ It strengthens abdominal organs, digestive system, excretory system.
- ➢ It helps in shedding extra belly fat.
- ➢ It helps in asthmatic condition and menstrual cramps.
- ➢ It soothes and relaxes mind.

PRECAUTIONS:

- ➢ Avoid this pose if you are suffering from backache, ulcer, knee pain, ankle injury, blood pressure problems, headaches and insomnia.

38. SIMHA ASANA

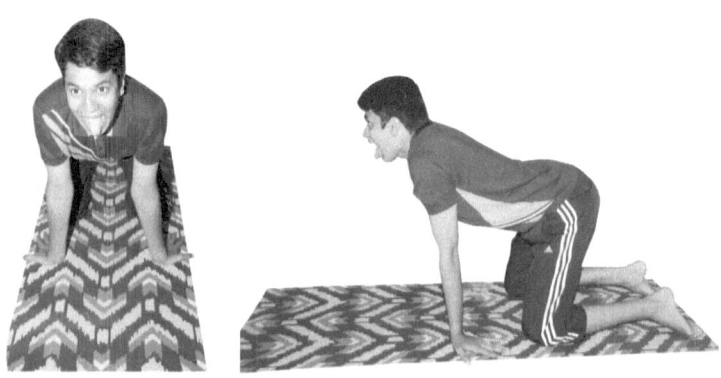

SIMHA=POWERFUL; ASANA= POSE

Steps:

- ❖ Sit down erect on the heels of the folded feet as shown in the picture.
- ❖ Rest the palms on the knees.
- ❖ Slightly lean forward, stretch the mouth jaws as wide as possible, take the tongue out of your mouth as much as you can and allow it to fall downward.
- ❖ Focus at the tip of nose.
- ❖ Stay in the pose as long as you can and then retract back your tongue in the mouth, close your mouth jaws.
- ❖ Release yourself to your relaxed pose.

BENEFITS:

- ➤ It tones and stretches muscles of various parts of face (jaw, mouth, throat, tongue)
- ➤ It relieves from sore throat.

PRECAUTIONS:

- ➤ It should be performed only under supervision and guidance of trained yoga teacher.

39. MAYUR ASANA

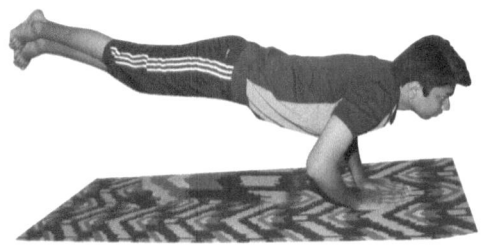

MAYUR=PEACOCK; ASANA= POSE

Steps:

- ❖ Lie down in the inverted pose such that face, abdomen, knees and foot toes should touch the floor with your straight hands lying on both sides on the floor.
- ❖ Now bend elbows and bring your palm just close to chest on the floor.
- ❖ Bend your right knee inward and fold your right leg in L shape and lift your left straight leg up in the air like peacock feathers, balancing on both palms and half right leg from knee to toe resting on the floor as shown in the picture.
- ❖ Now lift up your chest along your head as shown in picture.
- ❖ Stay in the pose as long as body allows.
- ❖ Now bring down your head, chest and left foot and straighten your right knee on the floor
- ❖ Now repeat with other side of feet.

BENEFITS:

> It stretches and strengthens the abdominal area, reproductive organs and the arm muscles.
> All vital organs are rejuvenated.
> It relieves from acidity, indigestion, diabetes, piles and constipation.
> It relaxes nerves and increases focus and concentration.

PRECAUTIONS:

> Avoid this pose during pregnancy and menstrual cycle and if one is suffering from any elbow, shoulder or wrist injury, hernia, ulcers, heart disease, blood pressure problems, brain tumour, intestinal problems, and eye, ear or nose infections.

40. TAAD ASANA

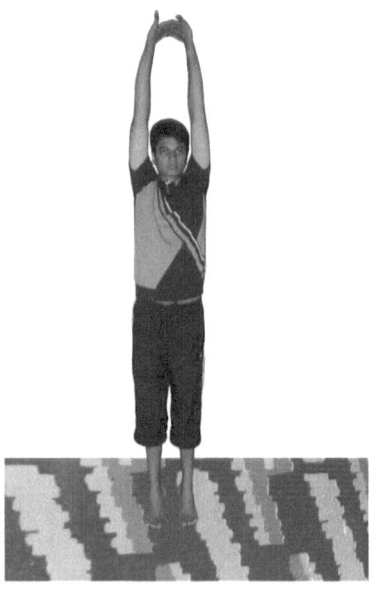

TAAD=PALM TREE; ASANA= POSTURE/POSE

Steps:

- ❖ Stand upright straight on the ground with a small gap between your feet.
- ❖ Raise both your arms while inhaling and keep them upwards by interlocking your fingers.

❖ Raise yourself on the toes as shown in the picture and feel the pressure of the stretch.

❖ Try to maintain this pose as long as you can with slow and deep breathing.

❖ Exhale and slowly lower down your arms and heels returning to your normal position.

BENEFITS:

➢ This is the only Asana to to increase the height of body.

➢ It soothes nerves and strengthens spinal cord and heart.

➢ It relieves from the indigestion.

PRECAUTIONS:

➢ Avoid it during pregnancy and if you are suffering from headaches, blood pressure problems and insomnia.

41. DANDA ASANA

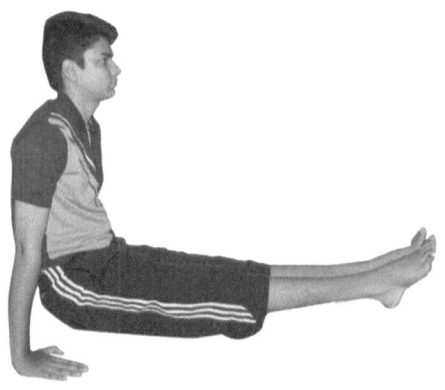

Danda=staff; Asana= Posture/Pose

Steps:

- ❖ Sit down with upright back with extended legs in front of you. Your legs and feet should be in straight line with hip.
- ❖ Rest your palms on your side on the floor.
- ❖ Now support your hip and raise your both feet upwards simultaneously as shown in the picture.
- ❖ Stay in the pose as long as body allows and then lower down your leg slowly.

BENEFITS:

> It enhances the flexibility of hips and pelvis.
> It improves the posture of lower back.

PRECAUTIONS:

> Avoid it during pregnancy and if you are suffering from headaches, blood pressure problems and insomnia.

42. KURMA ASANA

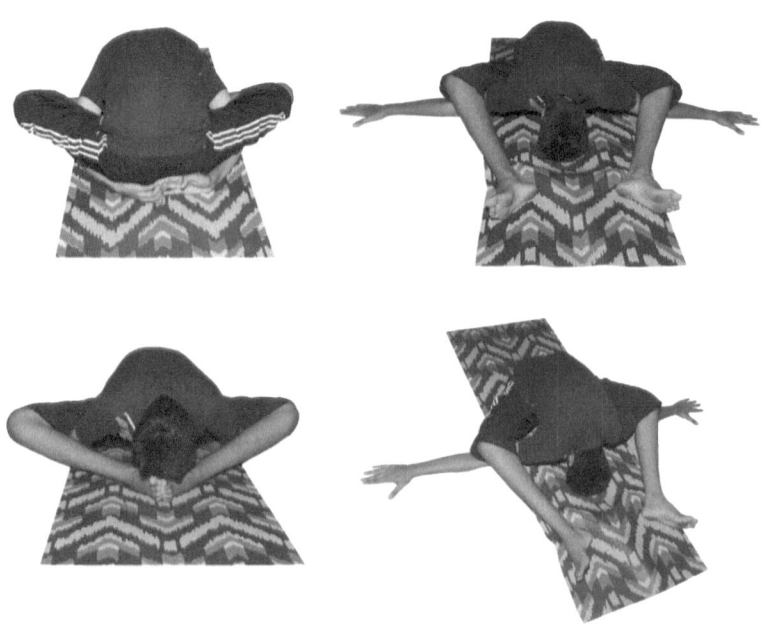

KURMA=TORTOISE; ASANA= POSE

Steps:

- ❖ Sit down with upright back with extended legs in front of you. Your legs and feet should be in straight line with hip.
- ❖ Rest your palms on your side on the floor.

❖ Now bend both knees from side and fold your legs inwards in such a way that soles of both legs meet each other.
❖ Now bend your upper part of body forward till your face reaches floor and spread both arms straight on your sides by passing them through from under bent knees.
❖ Your spread arms should be in straight line as shown in picture.
❖ Hold this position while breathing 3-8 times.

BENEFITS:

➢ It gives good stretching to back, leg and spine.
➢ It smoothens the functioning of the digestive and respiratory systems.
➢ It relaxes lumber and sacrum areas.
➢ It relaxes mind.

PRECAUTIONS:

➢ Avoid any force on the muscles during this asana.
➢ Avoid this asana if you are suffering from any arm, hip or shoulder injuries.

43. DWIPADA UTTANAPAD ASANA

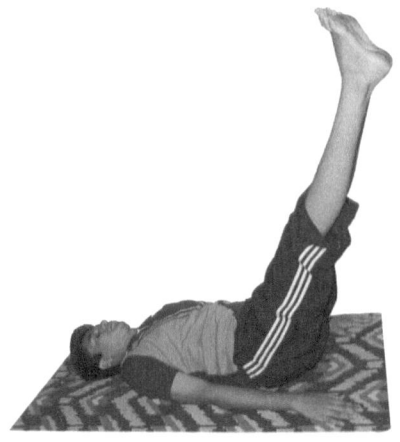

DWI=TWO, PADA=FEET, UTTAN=RAISED; ASANA= POSE

Steps:

- ❖ Lie down on the floor with whole body in straight line with your hands resting on both sides with palms touching the floor.
- ❖ Now lift both feet from hip upwards towards the sky as shown in the picture.
- ❖ Stay in the pose as long as you can and then lower down your legs to the floor without any jerk.

BENEFITS:

- ➢ It tones abdominal, thigh, pelvic and perineal muscles.
- ➢ It regulates the production of digestive juices and the process of excretion.
- ➢ It facilitates flow of carbon dioxide rich blood from the leg region towards the heart.

PRECAUTIONS:

- ➢ Avoid this asana if you have undergone any abdominal surgery.

44. PADANGUSTHA ASANA

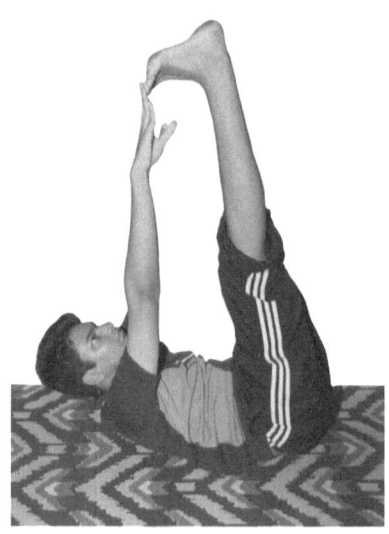

PADAN= FEET, ANGUSTHA = TOE; ASANA= POSTURE/POSE

Steps:

* ❖ Lie down on the floor with whole body in straight line with your hands resting on both sides with palms touching the floor.
* ❖ Now lift both feet from hip upwards towards the sky as shown in the picture.
* ❖ Now raise both hands straight upwards and try to hold toe of your raised feet as shown in the picture.

❖ Make sure do not allow to bend knees.
❖ Stay in the pose as long as your body allows and then bring down your legs and hands slowly without any jerk.

BENEFITS:

➢ It controls blood pressure and anxiety and improves focus and memory retention power.

PRECAUTIONS:

➢ Avoid this pose If you suffers from any back or neck injuries.

45. KARNAPIDASANA

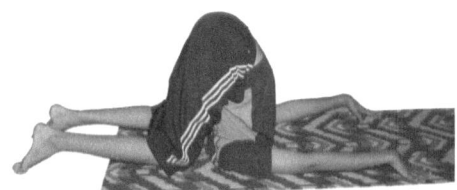 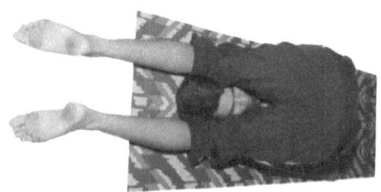

<small>KARNA=EAR, PIDA=PAIN; ASANA= POSTURE/POSE</small>

Steps:

- ❖ Lie down on the floor on your back in resting position with arms resting at the sides.
- ❖ Your legs should be straight in front of you.
- ❖ Inhale and keep down your palms in the floor.
- ❖ Now raise your legs in the air and try to exhale.
- ❖ Try to keep your legs erect in the air. (at 90 degree).
- ❖ Now place your legs over your head.
- ❖ Now try to lift up your butts and try to bend your legs over the head. (Bend or press your knee into the floor by your upper arms just near to ear, and try to press and place them just near to ear).
- ❖ Your arms should be parallel to our body.
- ❖ For supporting your hips, lift up your hands and keep them under your lower back.

❖ Try to grab your bend knees together.

❖ After that put down your knees and take a deep breath.

❖ Now lift up your butts and keep down your knees.

❖ After that open your bend knees and keep them on the ground.

❖ Now keep your legs on the ground and try to stretch your arms in parallel pose.

❖ Place your palms open over the floor facing towards the ceiling as shown in picture.

❖ Hold this position for around 6 to 8 breathes.

❖ At last keep down your arms in the floor and get back in the initial position and rest for a minute and repeat the process about 3 to 5 times.

BENEFITS:

➢ It stretches and strengthens hip, thighs, shoulder and spine.

➢ It is helpful in asthma, menopause, backache, infertility, sinusities.

➢ It relaxes whole body.

➢ It stimulates the smooth functioning of thyroid gland.

PRECAUTIONS:

➢ Avoid this pose in case of diarrhoea, menstrual cycle, neck injury and blood pressure problems.

46. GARUD ASANA

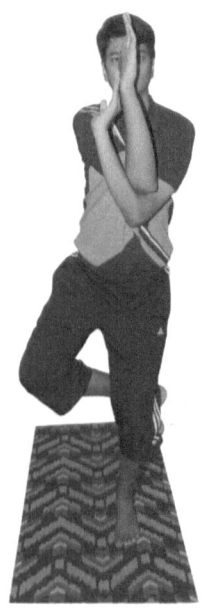

GARUD=BIRD (EAGLE); ASANA= POSE

Steps:

- ❖ Stand upright straight in erect position with hands down on your side.
- ❖ Open straight your palms.
- ❖ Bring your both arms in salutation pose by bending elbows.

❖ Make both arms from elbow till hand, parallel to each other with open stretched arms pointing towards sky.

❖ Now cross parallel portion of arm like embrace, keeping open stretched palm pointing upwards.

❖ Now firm your feet on the ground, and while maintaining balance on one foot lift other foot and embrace the calve muscles of the foot placed on the floor as shown in picture.

❖ Stay in the pose for a while and then release to normal standing relaxed pose.

BENEFITS:

➤ It improves balance and stretches your upper back, pelvis, shoulders and outer thighs.

➤ It strengthens legs, knees and ankles.

PRECAUTIONS:

➤ Avoid this pose if you are suffering from arm, hip or knee injury.

D. MEDITATION

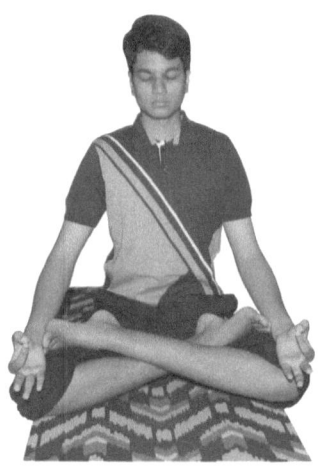

Meditation is that stage of body, in which it relaxes from deep inside. Meditation is often mistaken for intense concentration or focus but in reality it is the state of absolute relaxation of mind when mind is free from any clutter of thoughts.

In other words meditation is cleansing of mind. And a clean mind is source of energy which heals, relaxes and rejuvenates our physical body giving unconditional happiness.

So all those who wants unconditional happiness, meditation is the key.

- ❖ Meditation strengthens our decision making ability.
- ❖ It enhances our mental faculties.
- ❖ It instills self belief.
- ❖ It allows to respect self as well as to others.

E. PRANAYAM

"Prana"= Breath; "ayama"= control

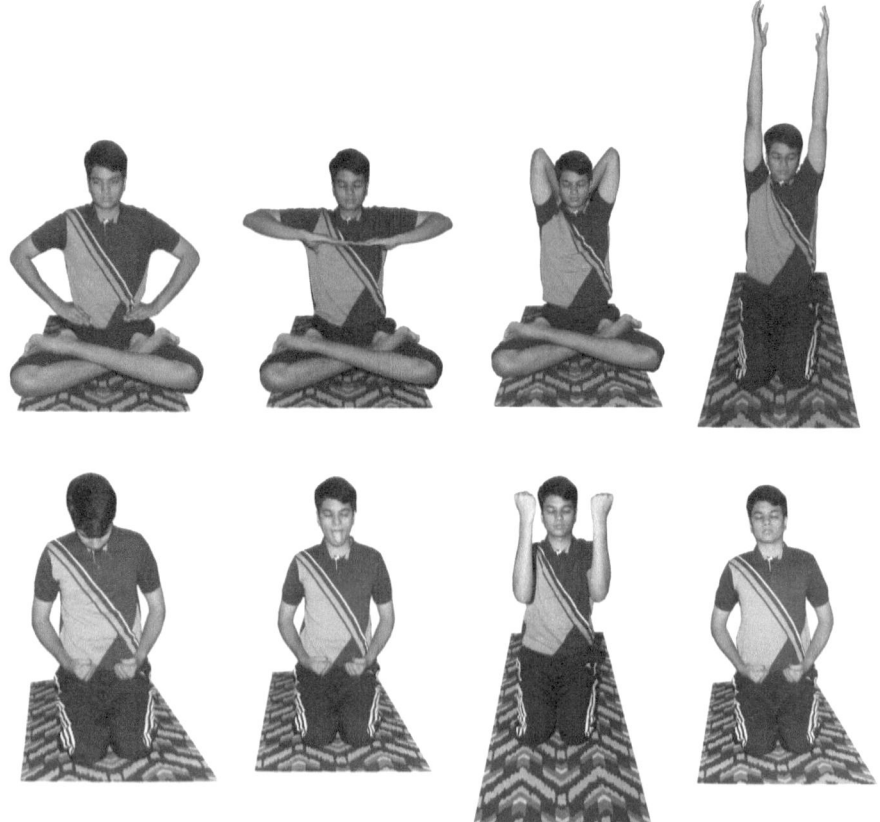

Prananyam is a technique by which we can control our breathing. Breathing is not simply inhaling and exhaling of air. But breathing means supply of oxygen to each cell of our body which is very important for each of our metabolic activities, and when we regulate this supply to each cell we ensures well coordinated functioning of all faculties of our body resulting healthy body and mind which is the root of unconditional happiness

TYPES OF PRANAYAMS (BREATHING)

1.	Fast Breathing
2.	Anulom Viloma
3.	Bhastrika Pranayam
4.	Kapalbhati
5.	Bhramari Pranayam

1. FAST BREATHING

Breathing involves two steps:

First- inhalation of air

Second exhalaltion of air.

Both the steps comprises one cycle of breathing.

When we breathe normally we do inhalation and exhalation without any conciousness.

In fast breathing, as the name suggests frequency of our cycle is increased upto 80-100 breaths/ minute.

BENEFITS:

> It gives exercise to all organs participating in respiration mechanism like diaphragm, coastal muscles, lungs and heart.
> It helps in low blood pressure.
> With every exhalation toxins are thrown out of body and when this exhalation is followed by inhalation, maximum toxins are removed before their remanufacturing resulting refreshing of each cell.
> It enables even to unclog blocked sinusitis.

PRECAUTIONS:

➢ Fast breathing should be avoided in pregnancy and as it increases blood pressure so high blood pressure patient should refrain from fast breathing.

➢ It should be done after consultation of medial expert if one is suffering from any disease.

➢ It is a prevention, not cure to any disease.

➢ If any one feels any inconvenience during fast breathing in terms of faintness, should stop fast breathing immediately and breathe normally.

2. ANULOMA-VILOMA

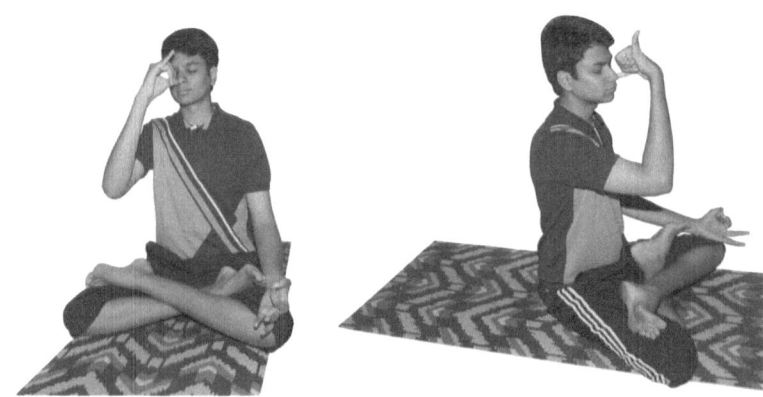

Steps:

- ❖ Anuloma – viloma is alternate nostril breathing.
- ❖ In this type of breathing, sit in padamasan.
- ❖ Now take out right hand, make a U with the thumb and ring finger.
- ❖ Now bring it close to nose as shown in the picture and press right nostril with thumb and inhale from left nostril.
- ❖ Now press left nostril with ring finger and remove thumb from right nostril.
- ❖ Exhale out from right nostril.
- ❖ Now inhale from right nostril and close this nostril with thumb and release ring finger from left nostril and exhale out.
- ❖ Continue this process.

BENEFITS:

> ➤ It allows more supply of oxygen to cells.
> ➤ It opens blockages in the nose related to sinusities.
> ➤ It calms mind.

PRECAUTIONS:

> ➤ It should be started with small number of breathing as comfortable to your body.
> ➤ With gradual practice it should be increased.
> ➤ Anyone who is surgically treated should consult medical practitioner before doing this breathing.

3. BHASTRIKA PRANAYAM

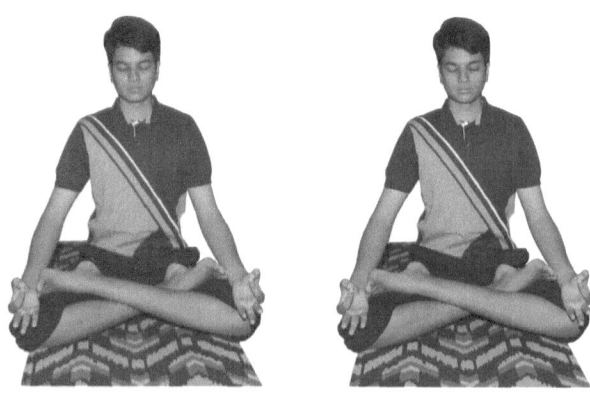

Bʜᴀsᴛʀɪᴋᴀ= ʙᴇʟʟᴏᴡs

Steps:

- ❖ Sit down erect in Padamasan.
- ❖ Now inhale from both nostrils as much as you can till you feel that diaphragm is pushed down.
- ❖ Now exhale out with full force through your nose till your diaphragm is pulled up.
- ❖ Keep your upper part of body upright during this process.
- ❖ Repeat as long as your body feels comfortable..

BENEFITS:

- ➤ It tones abdominal muscles and lungs.
- ➤ It throws away toxic very quickly thus cleaning system.
- ➤ It refreshes body and mind.
- ➤ It strengthens respiratory system.

PRECAUTIONS:

- ➤ Avoid in pregnancy, high blood pressure or any nervous disorder.
- ➤ It should be done empty stomach.

4. KAPALBHATI

Kapal=skull; Bhati=illuminating

Kapalbhati Pranayama is a breathing techniques that exert profound physiological effects on cardiovascular, and mind also.

Kapalabhati Pranayama needs breathe coordination at higher rate and thence, higher rate of metabolism muscle activity, that made strengthening of the metabolism muscles and resulted in improvement of respiratory organ operate. In Kapalbhati Pranayama we exhale with stroke. Most important point to remember, is that when you are exhale while doing Kapalbhati Pranayama assume that all the mental and physical disorder are kicked out from your body and mind also. Keep assuming that feeling in every stroke of exhale. It is the simple and easy to do Pranayam but having powerful effect.

Steps:

- ❖ Sit down straight in the Padmasana.
- ❖ Now inhale for long through nostrils till you feel no more air is going inside your nostrils.
- ❖ Now Exhale out with full force through nostrils itself till you feel no more air is coming from your nostrils and diaphragm is stretched upwards upto it's maximum limit.

❖ During forceful exhalation one may have some sound as air passes with speed.

❖ Repeat this process as long as your body allows you comfortably.

BENEFITS:

➤ It calms body and mind.

➤ It stimulates excretory system and circulatory system

➤ It gives glow on face and skin.

➤ It reduces dark circles around the eyes.

➤ It stimulates cardiovascular functioning.

PRECAUTION:

➤ Avoid it If one is suffering from acidity, ulcer, high blood pressure, cardiac problems.

5. BHRAMARI PRANAYAM
(Bee Breathe)

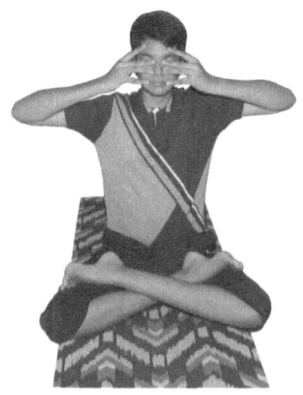

Steps:

❖ Sit down erect in the Padmasana.
❖ Now take thumbs of both hands and place them on the ear so as to cover ear hole.
❖ Now spread rest four fingers in such a way that index finger is above your eyebrows and remaining three fingers gently rests on your eye lids and side of your nose.
❖ Push last finger slightly which is just side of nose.
❖ Now breath in and while breathing out make sure mouth is closed so that while exhaling when you pronounce word

"Om", that sound vibrates in your mouth and transform into vibrating humming sound.

❖ You can feel vibration of humming sound on your face and within yourself.

BENEFITS:

➢ It is a stress buster exercise.
➢ It helps in cardiac problems, headaches and high blood pressure.
➢ It relaxes mind and brain.
➢ It is safe on all systems so can be done by anybody.
➢ It regulates the smooth functioning of the Endocrine system.

PRECAUTIONS:

➢ It should be done empty stomach.
➢ It is preferable if done after Anulom - vilom Pranayama
➢ Thumb and fingers should be gently placed on ear hole and eye lids.

F. POWER JOGGING

THIS IS SIMILAR TO JOGGING. JOGGING, COUPLED WITH SCIENTIFIC MEASURES, BECOMES HIGHLY EFFECTIVE AND REJUVENATING. POWER JOGGING IS COMBINATION OF TWELVE ACTIVITIES. THESE ACTIVITIES ARE IN CO-ORDINATION TO EACH OTHER. IT WARMS UP AND REJUVENATES BODY FOR DAILY ROUTINE ACTIVITIES.

Step 1: Ensure the following breathing pattern before you start –

- ◦ Inhale while bend right hand and right leg.
- ◦ Exhale while bending left side hand and leg.

- ❖ Relax and stand.
- ❖ Now run on the same place by deep breathing.
- ❖ While exhaling bring one clenched punch by bending elbow towards shoulder while another clenched fist should be straight close to the side of hip.
- ❖ While doing this bend knee in such a way that heel of bend leg should touch hip as shown in picture.

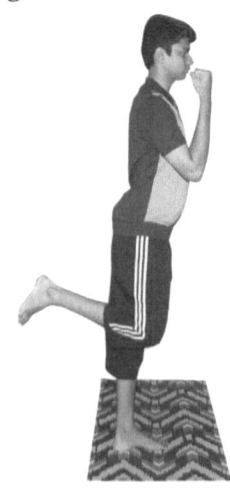

❖ Now during running on the same place repeat with other hand and leg similarly.

❖ Leg and hand will bend of same side.

❖ Repeat the cycle for 10-15 times with the fast pace.

Step 2: Ensure the following breathing pattern before you start –

    ◦ Inhale while bend right hand and right leg.

    ◦ Exhale while bending left side hand and leg.

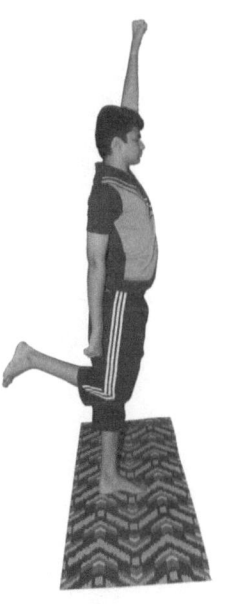

❖ Now do not bend elbow.

❖ While running on same place take your hand up by taking full half circle from front to back and then down close to hip anticlockwise circle as shown in picture.

❖ Leg action will remain same. Try to touch buttock with heel of back raised feet

❖ Like the step 1, once circular movement is completed repeat with other hand and leg.

❖ Repeat the cycle 10-15 times with fast pace.

Step 3: Continue with the same breathing pattern -

❖ Place both of your palm on your back...

❖ Jump and quickly inhale and bend one of your knee and try to touch knee with your chest.

❖ Now while exhaling bring down bent feet as shown in picture.

❖ Now again inhale and repeat with other feet.

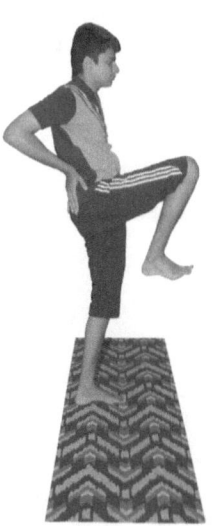

❖ Repeat the steps for 10-15 times with fast pace.

Step 4: Continue with the same breathing pattern -

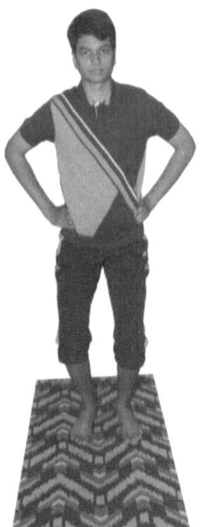

❖ Stand on toes shoulder width apart.
❖ Place both of your palm on your side back
❖ Now while exhaling keeping upper body straight, bend down on knees as low as you can maintain body balance as shown in picture.
❖ Similarly straighten up your knees and lift up your body while inhaling.
❖ Repeat the steps 10-15 times with fast pace.

Step 5: Continue with the same breathing pattern –

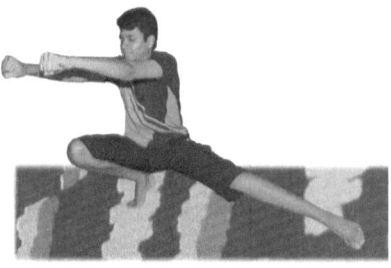

❖ Stand on toes with maximum distance apart.
❖ Now bring both hands in front of you parallel to ground as well as parallel to each other.
❖ While exhaling bend one knee and sit on toes of that feet keeping torso straight so that hip can rest on the heel of bent knee foot as shown in picture.

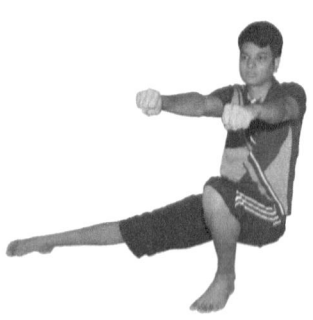

❖ Now while inhaling bring yourself in the centre.
❖ Repeat the same with other feet.
❖ Repeat the steps 10-15 time with fast pace.

Step 6: Continue with the same breathing pattern –

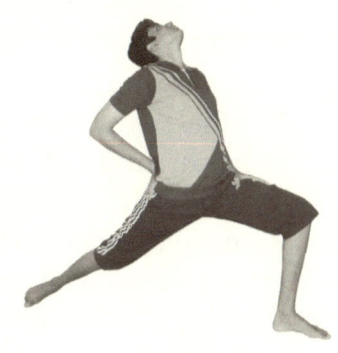

- ❖ Stand on toes with maximum distance apart.
- ❖ Place your palm on hips and stand straight.
- ❖ Move your upper body towards one toe and bend that knee and sit with the support of same foot.
- ❖ Keep upper torso straight.
- ❖ Back foot knee will not bend and remain straight touching the ground with toes only as shown in picture.

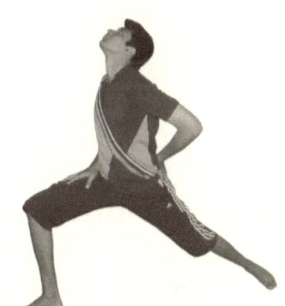

- ❖ Now come back to original position while exhaling.
- ❖ Repeat the same with other side.
- ❖ Repeat the steps 10-15 times with full pace.

Step 7: Continue with the same breathing pattern -

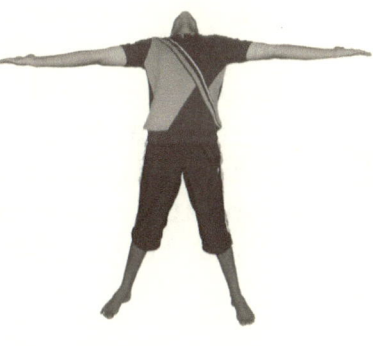

- ❖ Stand on toes with maximum distance apart
- ❖ Spread your hands straight in front of you parallel to ground.
- ❖ Now while inhaling take away your hands to back without tilting passing through sides.
- ❖ Chest and neck will bend backwards as shown in picture.
- ❖ Now while exhaling bring your hands front making chest and shoulder tilt forward.
- ❖ Inhale and repeat the cycle 10-15 times with full pace.

Step 8: Continue with the same breathing pattern -

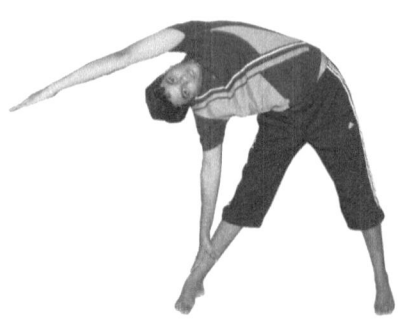

- ❖ Stand on toes with maximum distance apart
- ❖ Inhale and lift your one hand, make it pass cross your ear and head and move to other side as much as possible, while slide down palm of other hand on the feet as shown in the picture.
- ❖ Exhale and come to starting position.
- ❖ Repeat same with other side.
- ❖ Repeat the cycle 10-15 times with full pace.

Step 9: Continue with the same breathing pattern -

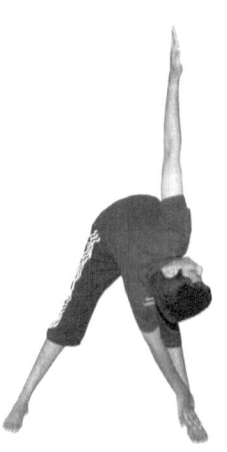

- ❖ Stand on toes with maximum distance apart
- ❖ Bend forward while exhaling and touch right foot with palm of right hand and second hand should point straight upwards.
- ❖ Gaze your upward hand pointing to sky as shown in the picture.
- ❖ Inhale and come to original position.
- ❖ Repeat the same with other side.
- ❖ Repeat the cycle 10-15 time with full pace.

Step 10: Continue with the same breathing pattern -

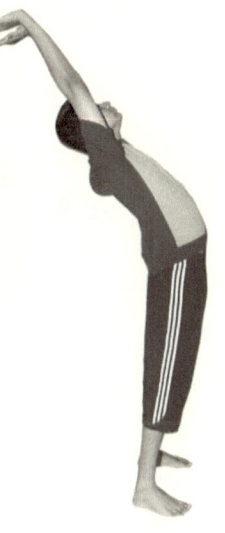

- ❖ Stand on toes with maximum distance apart
- ❖ Inhale and take both straight parallel hands upward towards sky and bend as much as you can. While doing so hands should touch your ears.
- ❖ Now while exhaling withy full pace bring forward your hand and without bending knee touch the front toe or ground.
- ❖ Try to touch forehead with knee as shown in the picture.
- ❖ Now inhale and come to original position.
- ❖ Repeat the cycle 10-15 times with full speed.

Step 11: Continue with the same breathing pattern –

- ❖ Stand on toes with maximum distance apart
- ❖ Inhale and lift your both hands from side.
- ❖ Take them upward and make a clap as shown in picture.
- ❖ Now exhale and jump and bring both hands down to side.
- ❖ Repeat the cycle 10-15 times with full speed.

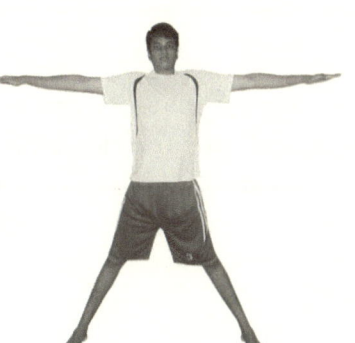

Step 12: Continue with the same breathing pattern -

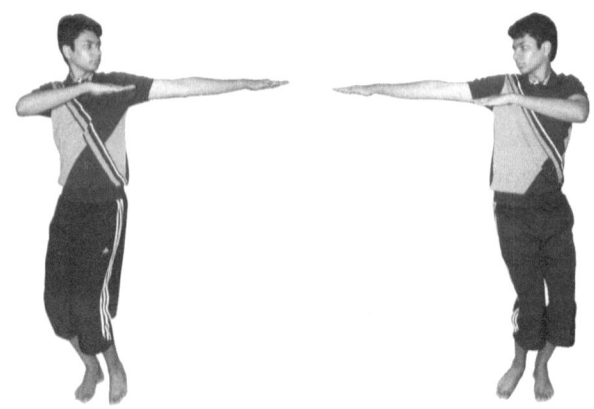

> Stand on toes with least distance apart
> Spread your hands straight in front of you parallel to ground
> Now jump in this way that back, knee and toe is in one direction and both parallel hands in other direction as shown in picture.
> Inhale when back is in right side and hands are in left side and exhale when back and exhale when back is in left side and hands are in right side.
> Repeat with full speed.
> Repeat the cycle 10-15 time with full pace.
> Neck and hand will face in the direction of hand.

BENEFITS:

> Your body becomes active and healthy.
> It gives strength and flexibility to body.
> It helps in strengthening of bones and joints.
> It refreshes and rejuvenates whole body.

PRECAUTIONS:

> - It can be done both times morning as well as evening.
> - It should be done empty stomach.
> - Diligent precaution of inhaling and exhaling during exercise gives maximum benefit.

G. SERVICE IN COMMUNITY

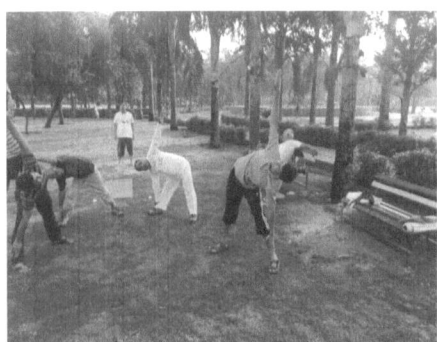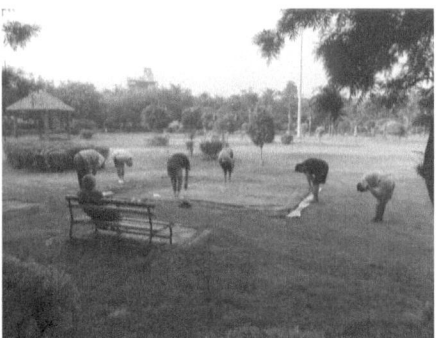

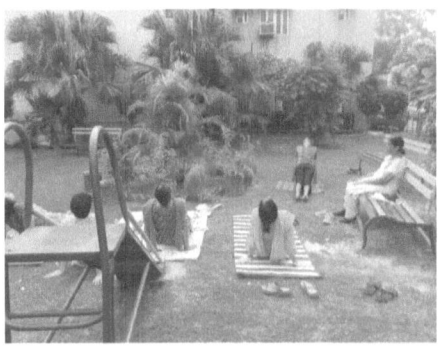

I have realized that for contribution to my community, it's not necessary for an NGO or Government to take an initiative. I can contribute to it on my own also. Our community is filled with healthy (and I am not talking about the good healthy) and people with laid back lifestyle, who seem to lack the motivation to take the first step in keeping themselves fit. Most of us seem to struggle to achieve a work-life balance.

I have been practicing yoga for some time now and I can definitely feel an immense difference between the past me to the new me. And I want the same thing to be experienced by others. It has helped me to discard the accumulated negative, wasted and unwanted elements in my life thereby clearing my otherwise-cluttered schedule. The thing I love about Yoga is its flexibility – it can be done anywhere and does not require any additional equipment. Gathering yoga enthusiasts having no age bar, I always look forward to taking those free sessions on Sundays. We might meet once a week, but I enjoy these sessions immensely not only due to Yoga but also because I can share my ideas, contemplate on random information and have fun in general.

Summary ...

Yoga Asanas are extended form of physical exercises. They ensures smooth functioning of various systems (muscular system, skeletal system, digestive system, excretory system, respiratory system, nervous system and cardiovascular system). In this way Yoga is insurance to sound health. And sound health means peace and calmness which leads to unconditional happiness. In this book. I'll be guiding you through the important Asanas and Pranayama.

Remember, Yoga is about progression with patience, not perfection. Keep practicing and you will slowly perfect your postures, calm your mind, approach happiness and this book will be your friend along the way.

To A Happier You,
Manan Aggarwal

Please feel free to contact Manan
at his email at
Mananaggarwal99@gmail.com
for free classes.
Sundays – from 6AM to 8AM

www.ingramcontent.com/pod-product-compliance
Lightning Source LLC
Chambersburg PA
CBHW020519290526
45786CB00002B/671